THE TV VET BOOK
FOR STOCK FARMERS No. 1

£2.50

THE TV VET BOOK
FOR STOCK FARMERS No. 1

Recognition and Treatment
of Common Cattle Ailments

By
THE TV VET

FARMING PRESS LIMITED
FENTON HOUSE WHARFEDALE ROAD IPSWICH SUFFOLK

FIRST PUBLISHED 1964
SECOND EDITION (Completely Revised) 1970
THIRD EDITION (Revised) 1972
SECOND IMPRESSION (with amendments) 1974

Filmset and Printed Offset Litho by
Cox & Wyman Ltd, London, Fakenham and Reading

ISBN 0 85236 032 0

Contents

Foreword

By W. T. PRICE, C.B.E., M.C., B.Sc., A.R.I.C.S.
Past Principal of Harper Adams Agricultural College

THE author, one of our leading veterinary scientists, is a practising veterinary surgeon and has established in Staffordshire an Animal Hospital which is quite unique in its conception and action and is doing excellent work.

As the TV Vet he has made many appearances on television, broadcast programmes, and contributed numerous articles on a variety of vet subjects to the technical and popular press.

In preparing this book he has adopted a most original and clever presentation by putting the emphasis on photographs and illustrations rather than relying mainly on the written matter. In a book of 176 pages there are over 300 illustrations which put over his story in a simple but concise manner.

To the reader one good photograph will give a clear idea which might take some 20 pages of explanation in the text.

The common ailments in cattle are dealt with in sections which makes for easy reference, and the author starts off with Metabolic Diseases, then Conditions of the Skin, the Eyes, the Mouth, the Lungs, followed by sections on Husk, the Stomach, Johne's Disease, the Udder, the conditions of the Feet, and a final section on the General Handling of animals, which is a most important chapter.

Throughout he has stressed the need for good housing, sound nutrition and efficient management for the maintenance of good health and the prevention of disease.

Practical methods of diagnosis are given for the assessment of ailments when they occur, together with simple remedies and treatment, but the author is very careful to enumerate those conditions of ill-health and disease which necessitate the *immediate* calling in of expert advice.

To sum up, this book is a very informative and comprehensive work, presented in a novel and easy style to read, and should prove of much value and help to farmers and all those concerned in animal welfare. It should be a 'must', to be included on the farm bookshelf for current reading as well as reference.

W. T. PRICE

Newport,
Shropshire

Author's Preface

EVER since my student days I have been of the opinion that textbooks are cluttered up with irrelevant detail. Invariably they are written in complicated so-called 'technical' language which saps one's concentration and often literally drives one mad in desperate efforts at true understanding.

I have noticed also that, in these textbooks, illustrations are in the main few and far between, and are usually sited several pages away from the condition they depict.

In this book I have tried my utmost to eliminate both these faults. I have tried to stick to essential facts. I have tried to use language which everyone can follow and understand easily, and wherever possible I have used a picture to tell its own story alongside the written words.

I believe that, provided costs can be kept rational, all books of the future will be presented in this way. Every teacher now knows the value of visual aids and to my mind it is inevitable that this very true knowledge will be translated into textbooks. If this book can at least encourage others to try the same technique, then I'm sure the publishers and I will be well satisfied.

Although simple, the facts are nonetheless up to the standards of the latest knowledge. This makes the book not only suitable for all lay readers, but also for agricultural and veterinary students at the various colleges, and universities and—dare I say it—for veterinary surgeons also, especially those who want to refresh their memories literally at a glance without spending hours delving into huge tomes.

I would like to acknowledge the close co-operation of my photographer, Mr. George Pringle, who is well known in agricultural journalism and is responsible for the majority of the pictures in this book.

METABOLIC DISORDERS

1
Acetonaemia

IN all cases of acetonaemia there occurs what we call a hypoglycaemia, that is, a shortage of a simple sugar called glycogen in the cow's liver, muscles and blood. This shortage can be produced in several ways. In other words, acetonaemia is not always a disease in itself, but may be a symptom of a disease or a symptom of a disfunction.

In fact, any liver condition such as fluke, abscess, or tuberculosis can produce acetonaemia; as can also general debilitating diseases like pneumonia, metritis (inflammation of the womb) and mastitis.

However, in normal years and in the vast majority of cases acetonaemia is basically a digestive problem; and though, naturally enough, many conflicting theories have been put forward as to its precise cause, I shall stick to the essential accepted facts which I think form a rational explanation.

All cows have very low reserves of energy, and this is stored in the form of glycogen in the liver and muscles. They derive most of their energy from three digestive products which we call fatty acids. They are acetic acid, propionic acid and butyric acid. These fatty acids are formed inside the cow's first

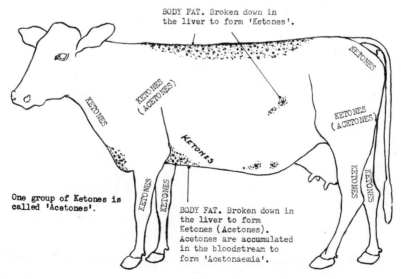

BODY FAT. Broken down in the liver to form 'Ketones'.

One group of Ketones is called 'Acetones'.

BODY FAT. Broken down in the liver to form Ketones (Acetones). Acetones are accumulated in the bloodstream to form 'Acetonaemia'.

13

stomach (the rumen), and from these acids the cows replenish their reserves of the simple sugar glycogen. They can, of course, utilise in a similar way other simple sugars like glucose.

When the energy demand becomes really high, as in peak milk production, the total energy required may be more than the food can provide. This causes the hypoglycaemia or deficiency of sugar in the blood. The cows then draw on the reserves in the liver and muscles.

Since these reserves are very low they are soon used up, and the cows have to turn to and draw on their stored body fat for the production of the extra energy which is still constantly required to keep up the milk production.

When this stored body fat is being broken down for energy (and the break-down occurs in the liver) certain substances which we call ketone bodies are formed and these ketones accumulate in the blood to produce the typical associated breath-smell.

One group of the ketone bodies is called acetones; hence the name aceto-naemia.

The hypoglycaemia, or reduced blood sugar level, together with the increased acetone concentration, causes a poisonous reaction in the affected cow and makes her dull and dopey, off her food and constipated. Naturally the milk yield drops immediately, which is nature's way of curing the condition, because as the milk yield drops so also does the energy demand of the body.

During the past few years it has been discovered that certain hormones play an important part in converting the fatty acids into blood sugar. These hormones are produced from a small gland at the base of the cow's brain—a gland called the pituitary—and also from two glands alongside the kidneys called the adrenal glands.

Hormonal research is still incomplete, and if I attempted to describe how the hormones work I am quite sure I would confuse everybody, including myself. So I think it is sufficient to establish that hormones are concerned and that synthetic hormones can be used successfully in treating acetonaemia.

Where It All Starts

Despite the fact that typical acetonaemic symptoms usually coincide with peak milk production round about a month after calving, the accumulation of the acetones may start during the last eight weeks of pregnancy. We must never forget this because it is important in prevention.

When acetonaemia is associated with high yields, it occurs chiefly in mature cows with a third, fourth or later calf, but second calvers can also get it, and I have actually seen one or two heifers with it. The animal in the pictures—a heifer— is suffering from the disease. Roughly one dairy cow in every hundred gets acetonaemia during the winter.

Symptoms

The first sign in cattle is loss of appetite. The cow is dull, and though she will eat hay, she usually refuses her concentrates.

Her breath has the characteristic sweet smell of acetones. The smell is quite distinctive and diagnostic (1). In fact, veterinary surgeons can often spot it as soon as they go into a cowshed.

When the patient goes off her food, naturally the milk yield drops. Not only is the milk less in quantity but it often reeks of acetones (2). The presence of the acetones can be confirmed by a simple milk test.

The cow's temperature is normal but she is constipated and the dung is often coated with slime (3). The stomach movements are sluggish and the patient quickly loses condition.

Occasionally a cow can develop a nervous acetonaemia and the symptoms of this are not unlike those of hypomagnesaemia. There is blindness, shiver-

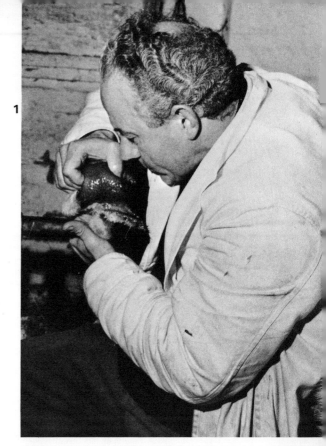

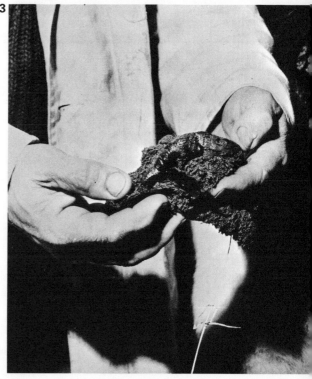

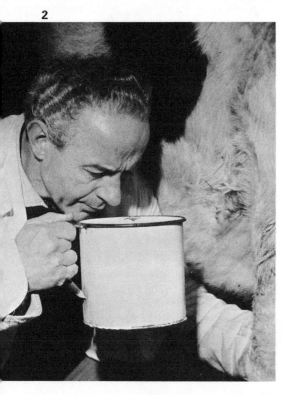

ing, hyper-excitability, and a mad type of uncontrollable licking.

Treatment

There are many treatments for acetonaemia, but obviously the most logical one comprises intravenous injection of simple sugars combined with drenches of a laxative like treacle mixed with glucose,

15

glycerol or a substance called sodium propionate (4). The sodium propionate changes into propionic acid in the rumen and the propionic acid is one of the chief sources of glycogen.

Apart from medicinal treatment, I usually advise stopping milking for 48 hours, part milking only for the following four or five days, and then gradually returning to full production.

Hormone injections, of course, are popular and often give spectacular results. They are injected straight into a muscle (5).

Prevention

But whichever way we may look at it, acetonaemia is expensive. The milk goes, the money goes, and the records are often ruined. So once again this is a disease which should be avoided if at all possible. Though the problem will vary slightly from farm to farm, the main point I want to make is that acetonaemia can be prevented by making use of intelligent

4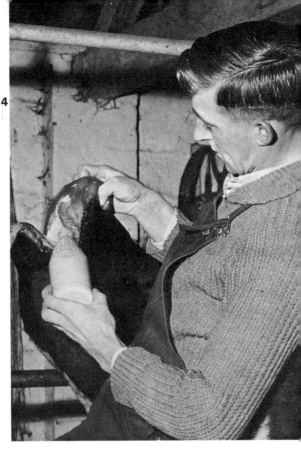

5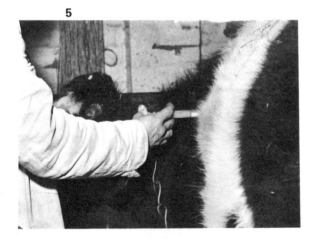

husbandry methods based on the simple facts we have established above.

To my mind careful feeding is the answer—remember acetonaemia can start at any time within the last two months of pregnancy. During that time excess energy is required to cope with the final development of the calf, and if the cow is not properly fed it will turn to its body fat and trigger off the disease.

There should always be adequate protein and carbohydrate in the diet of the dry cow, but even more important is an ample sufficiency of fibre, preferably in the form of good hay. Remember, the bulk of the energy is produced in the cow's first stomach, and the fibre is essential to keep the concentrates in the rumen long enough to allow the breakdown of the food to the fatty acids. Self-feed silage usually provides sufficient fibre, though sometimes hay is needed to balance the fibre content. Personally, when I am investigating an acetonaemic outbreak I always insist on at least a part diet of hay (6).

After calving the fibre and carbohydrate should be maintained at the same level and this is probably just as important as the pre-natal feeding.

The protein push towards the high yields should never be forced, but should

be done very gradually during the first six **6**
weeks of lactation. In other words, aim
to get the peak yield at six weeks rather
than at four.

If you are troubled with acetonaemia,
then it will pay handsomely throughout
this vital 14-week period to use compound
concentrates of a high grade, and to feed
these often in comparatively small quantities. Purchased compounds are preferable
to home-grown mixtures because they are
more likely to provide a better balance of
readily assimilable food (7).

Feeding glucose in the form of powder
or blocks throughout this 14-week period
can be very valuable, but to my mind this
is just a substitute for good husbandry (8).

Just one last simple preventive measure
—exercise. If your cows are not in open
yards, they should be turned out for at
least an hour every day. As with us,
exercise promotes healthy digestion, and
to the pregnant or milking cow a healthy
digestion is the most valuable of all assets.

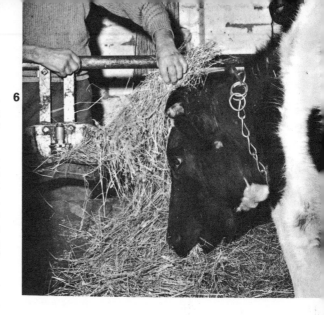

8

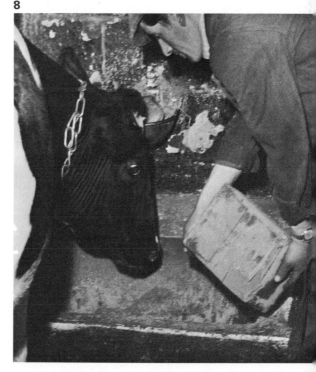

7

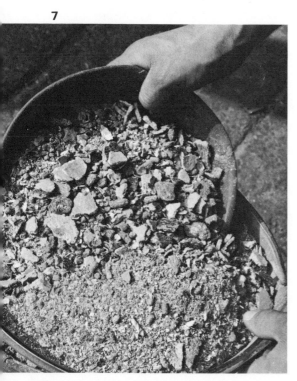

17

2
Aphosphorosis

THE term aphosphorosis means simply a deficiency of the mineral phosphorus in the blood of an affected animal.

Cause
It is caused either by a straightforward deficiency in the feed or pasture or by an upset in the blood balance of phosphorus in relation to calcium magnesium and vitamin D.

How It Produces Its Effect
Phosphorus deficiency upsets the filtration mechanism of the kidneys and produces an oedema or dropsy of that area. This oedema causes a paralysis of the hindquarters. Mild phosphorus deficiency occasionally causes 'pica', *i.e.,* a perverted appetite which may make the affected animals show a craving for such things as the bark of trees.

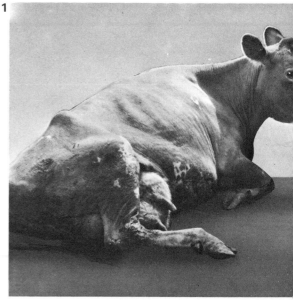

How To Recognise It
The mild cases of pica are often difficult or impossible to detect but in the more acute cases the affected animals are found down and unable to rise (1). They may eat and behave perfectly normally otherwise. It is my experience that aphosphorosis affects chiefly in-calf cows during the last month of pregnancy. In fact whenever I have a cow down before calving I always treat it as a suspect asphosphorosis.

This is the condition which our forefathers in many parts of the country used to describe as 'the loin-drop'.

What To Do
Send for your veterinary surgeon. Don't, whatever you do, be tempted to try the

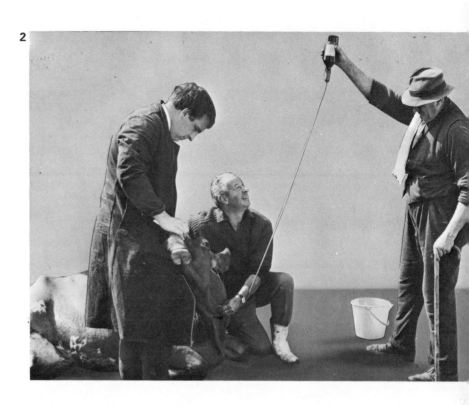

2

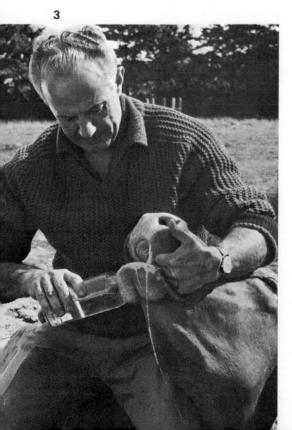

3

long outdated practice of applying mustard plasters to the cow's back.

The veterinary surgeon will inject concentrated phosphorus solution intravenously (2). In addition to the concentrated phosphorus, he may give a mixture of calcium, phosphorus and magnesium to take care of any possible upset in the mineral balance.

It is unwise to try injecting phosphorus intravenously on your own because if even a drop or two of the concentrated phosphorus solution gets under the cow's skin the resultant swelling and abscess can well nigh ruin her.

How Long a Cow Takes To Get Better

It is my experience that aphosphorosis cases may take 24 hours or longer to respond to treatment.

Occasionally the patients are down for several days. In such cases in addition to

19

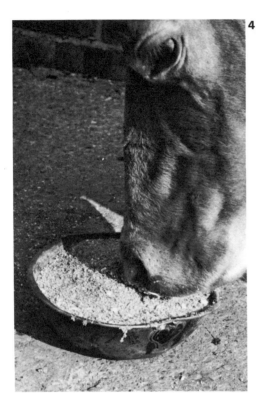

4

all the usual nursing precautions (hobbling, gritting, bedding, etc.) phosphorus should be given as a drench once daily (3). Again the veterinary surgeon should prescribe the drug and the dose.

How To Prevent It

Apparently it can be prevented to a very large extent by feeding foodstuffs rich in phosphorus, *e.g.,* kale or bran (4).

Another wise precaution, which helps a great deal, is to use basic slag on the pastures and the best time to sow this is in the winter around December or early January.

Aphosphorosis can manifest itself in other ways, *e.g.,* in the lack of bony growth in the calves, in a disappointing milk yield of the dairy cows, but most important of all, in infertility. Whenever there is difficulty in getting dairy cows to settle to the bull, therefore, the possibility of aphosphorosis should always be explored. Here (5) an examination for pregnancy is being carried out.

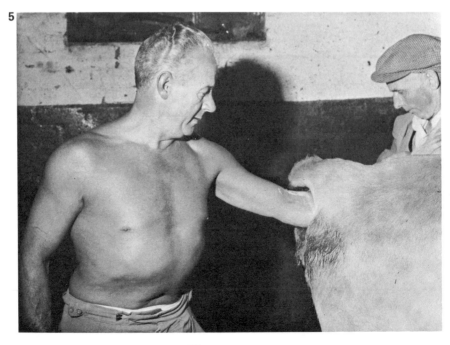

5

3
Hypomagnesaemia
(Grass Tetany or Grass Staggers)

HYPOMAGNESAEMIA means simply a deficiency of magnesium in the blood.

How Deficiency Occurs

In all ruminants, magnesium helps to control the action of the muscles. Since this function is very important the cow's body carries magnesium reserves. These magnesium reserves are stored on the surface of the crystalline framework of the bones, especially the rib bones and the vertebrae (1).

In young animals the bony framework is open. This means that the magnesium reserves are readily available and last for 40 to 50 days.

In older animals, where the bone structure is much more compact, the reserves don't last nearly so long. In fact, in the adult cattle the magnesium reserves may keep them going for no more than four or five days. This explains why the disease is more common in old cattle than in young ones.

It Can Affect Young Cattle

Hypomagnesaemia does occur in young cattle, but much less frequently and only when the diet has been short of magnesium for some time. It is occasionally seen in calves fed chiefly on cow's milk (2) with little or no access to hay. This is because the magnesium content of cow's milk is scanty and is certainly insufficient for the growing calves.

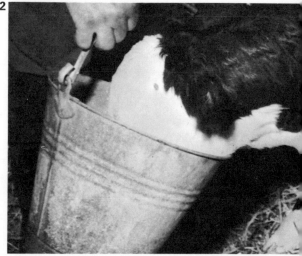

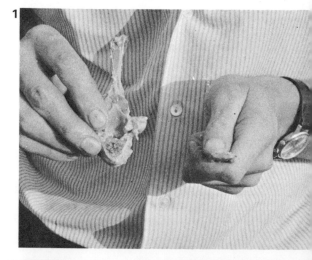

This explains another feature of the disease, *viz.,* why it is seen in beef calves three to four months old more often than in dairy calves. This is simply because beef calves are mostly suckled on the cow and are often given practically no supplementary food (3).

In some beef herds hypomagnesaemia affects chiefly the out-wintered, pregnant or lactating cows and it often flares up during a sudden cold spell.

In all herds, however, there is a gradual natural decline in magnesium reserves throughout the winter and all the cattle are lowest in magnesium in the spring round about turning out time.

If the herd is turned out on to a mature permanent pasture of normal seasonal growth, then any magnesium shortage in most cases is soon made good. Permanent grass tends to build up a reserve of soluble magnesium in the top soil and under normal conditions both the grass and the animals can utilise this.

If, however, the herd is turned out on to a young rapidly growing pasture which owes its early growth to the pasture application of artificial fertilisers, the story is different. Then it appears that either the artificials (especially sulphate of ammonia) hinder the plant uptake of magnesium or that the high nitrogen content of the young grass inhibits magnesium absorption in the animal's digestive tract. After four or five days of grazing on such pastures (in some cases after only a few hours) some of the older animals may develop hypomagnesaemia—hence the name grass tetany or grass staggers.

Symptoms

The symptoms are unmistakable—the patient starts to shiver violently, stagger wildly and unless treated quickly falls down in a fit, kicking and frothing at the mouth (4).

Symptoms like these may appear during the autumn and winter. In such cases the condition is triggered off by the hay or silage having been made early from

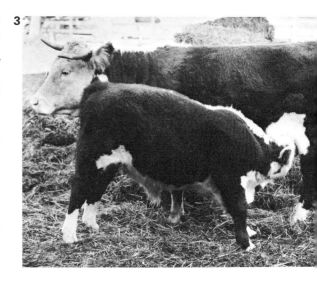

artificially stimulated grasses, or, in beef herds, by a sudden cold spell when the animals are already on a low plane of nutrition.

How To Control and Prevent Hypomagnesaemia

If the symptoms appear during the autumn or winter, then magnesium has to be fed. A daily ration of magnesium oxide—2 oz.

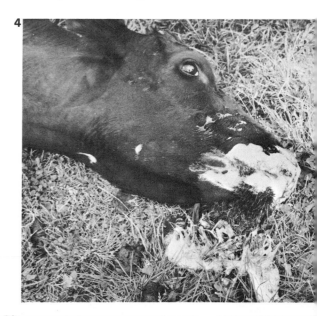

22

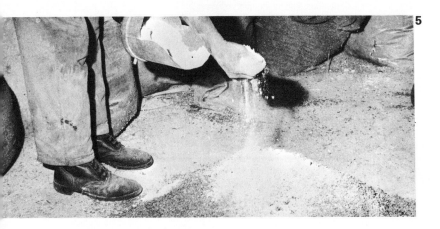

5

per head per day—should be fed to the entire herd. The cheapest concentrated source of magnesium oxide is a product called calcined magnesite. Calcined magnesite is unpalatable and therefore it has to be mixed very thoroughly with the feed. It is my experience that all cattle will eat it best when it is fed in wet beet pulp (5).

Feeding calcined magnesite can be used as a preventative at turning out time but, if so, feed-supplementation has to start at least 14 days before grazing and it has to continue right on to the end of June.

Where hypomagnesaemia is a major problem, the progressive farmer, in addi-

tion to feeding magnesium, may have to temper his use of artificial manures. He may also have to make at least a percentage of his hay or silage later from the more matured grasses.

Not only so, but he may have to reserve some untreated permanent pasture for the early grazing or at least daily alternate between the lush and the older grasses.

At all times he should strive to increase economically the magnesium content of his soil and pasture. The best way to do this is to use, as a routine, magnesian limestone instead of ordinary lime, but to be effective the magnesian limestone must contain at least 10% of magnesium (6).

6

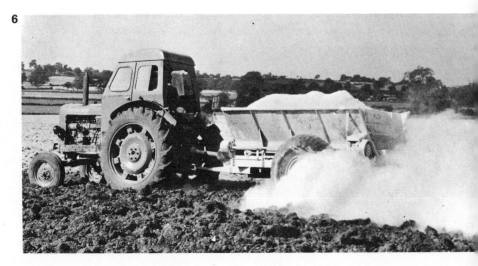

4
Milk Fever

MILK FEVER occurs chiefly in older cows and the symptoms generally appear during the first 24 hours after calving.

Cause

The condition is associated with a hypocalcaemia, which is a deficiency of calcium in the bloodstream. But the precise cause or trigger factor which produces this deficiency is as yet not completely understood.

The demand for calcium arises first of all during the growth of the calf within the cow. Considerable amounts are required for the build-up of the calf's bones and teeth, especially during the latter part of pregnancy. An excess of calcium is again required when the udder fills up with milk and colostrum immediately after calving.

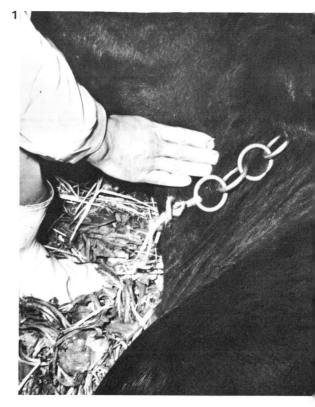

The theories concerning possible trigger factors are that milk fever can be due to:

(1) *Disfunction of the parathyroid glands.* These are the two small glands, situated in the neck (1). These supply the hormones that control the blood calcium concentration. The hormones cannot cope with sudden drastic changes in the blood calcium but require time to adapt themselves to the demands—with the result that the deficiency symptoms occur.

(2) *The age factor.* As the cow gets older the bones become hard, and the calcium reserves in the bones, which are very considerable, become less accessible to the bloodstream. This point is obvious if one studies a bone from an old cow (2). The

theory is borne out by the fact that 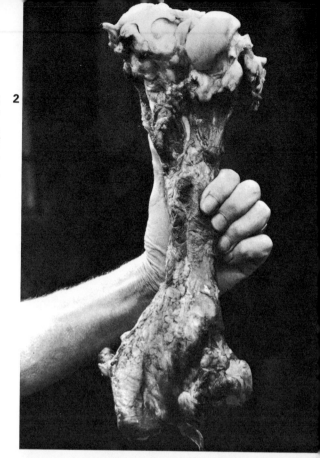 typical milk fever does not usually occur until the third, fourth or fifth calf. I have, however, seen first-calf heifers with it, and it is not uncommon in high-yielding second calvers.

(3) *Digestive disturbances.* Any digestive disturbance can lead to an upset in the absorption of calcium from the bowel. Certainly such disturbances can produce genuine hypocalcaemia because typical symptoms occur when the cow has gorged herself on concentrated feedingstuffs, not only on high-protein meals and cakes but also on any foodstuffs—even barley, oats or wheat. It can also occur in the spring when the cows are turned out on to lush grass, and it is an outstanding feature when sugar-beet tops, kale, potatoes or mangolds are fed to excess.

(4) *Shortage of calcium in the diet.*

(5) *A stress factor.* A severe milk fever can flare up after a long journey by road or rail. This condition is described as transit or transport tetany but nonetheless it is a genuine hypocalcaemia brought about apparently by the stress and strain of the journey.

Symptoms

The first sign is that the cow goes off her feed; usually she stops eating altogether. The ears are cold to the touch (3).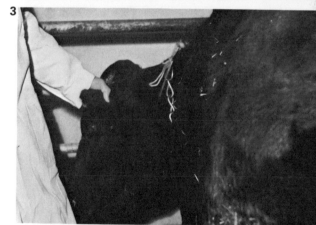

If untreated the patient may start to shiver and at the same time move the hind feet tentatively stiffening the hind legs alternately and weaving unsteadily from one to the other.

The temperature is normal (4) and the 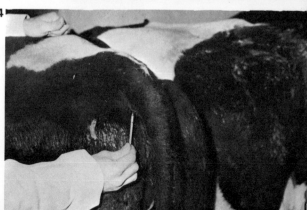 cow is usually constipated.

Within an hour or so the cow starts to breathe heavily and stagger about and very soon she flops down on one side. At this stage if she is sat up on her brisket she will either turn her head around and hold it tightly along her chest or she will hold it forward uncertainly with the neck in an S-shaped bend (5).

If still untreated the patient will start to throw herself about often injuring her head. After a few hours of this she becomes comatose.

Treatment
First and foremost, if the cow is tied up by a neck chain, always tie the chain with a link of string in case the staggering cow should flop down and hang herself. This is common sense.

Secondly, 'hobble' the hind legs, *i.e.,* tie them together above the fetlocks as illustrated (6). This will prevent the cow 'splaying' and thereby damaging her hips or pelvis. It is my experience that the usual cause of a milk fever cow not getting up after treatment is hip or pelvic damage caused either when the cow first goes down or when she is plunging about trying to stand up.

Thirdly, sprinkle sawdust, sand or grit underneath the affected animal's hind feet (7). This again will prevent her slipping about and injuring her legs and will also make it much easier for her to stand again if and when she goes down.

If, as often happens, a cow is found flat out and blown up first thing in the morning, then the best thing to do is to roll her on to her back (8) and over on to her brisket (9). *If this is not done quickly, in many cases the cow may die from bloat—caused by paralysis of the stomach muscles. In fact, practically all milk fever deaths are due to suffocation caused by the bloated and distended rumen pressing on the cow's diaphragm.*

If the bloat is excessive, emergency puncture may be necessary (*see* Bloat).

It is always well worthwhile sending for the veterinary surgeon to treat a milk fever case. There is a considerable chance that the deficiency may not be one of calcium but may be one of phosphorus or magnesium, neither of which would respond to straight calcium injections.

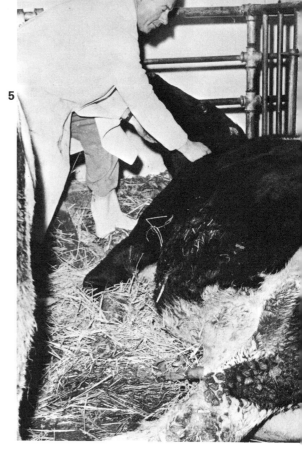

Not only so but milk fever symptoms can appear in other conditions, *e.g.,* gangrene of the udder. The conscientious veterinary surgeon will always check for this before making a diagnosis (10).

The injection of large amounts of calcium underneath the skin, although it

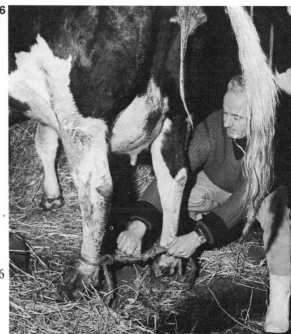

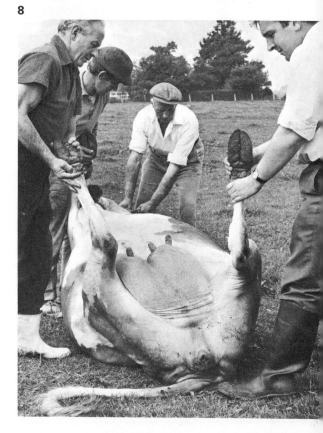

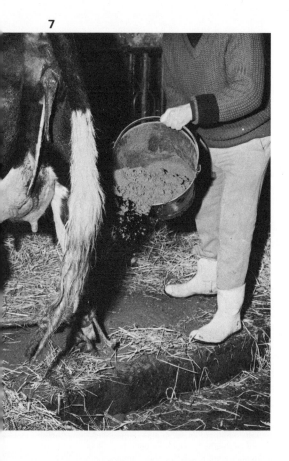

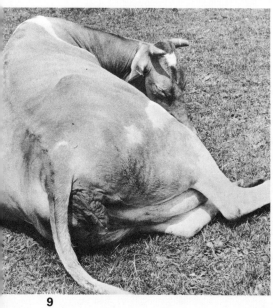

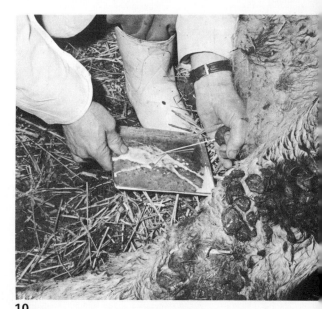

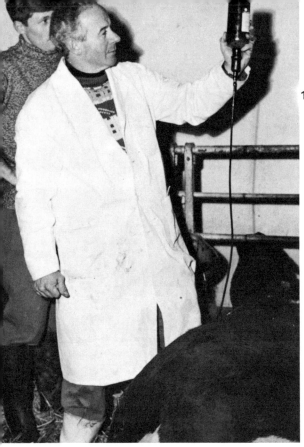

11 appears easy (11), requires a fair amount of skill if unsightly lumps and abscesses are to be avoided.

The administration of calcium intravenously can be especially dangerous because if the calcium is allowed to flow too rapidly it can damage the heart muscle and produce heart failure (12–13).

When the animal is down for several days good nursing is the vital factor if she is to survive. Adequate bedding, repeated turning and constant propping up on the brisket will prevent bed sores and make all the difference to the chances of complete recovery. In such cases the hind leg hobbling (14) and the sand or grit underneath the bedding are even more important (15).

Prevention

The danger period is the first 24 hours after calving, and practical prevention must be aimed at tiding the cow over this vital time. I would say, therefore, that the sensible thing to do on any farm where milk fever is common is to have each cow, from the third calf onwards, injected with calcium (16) as soon as she calves. It is my experience that there is little or no value in injecting before calving.

12

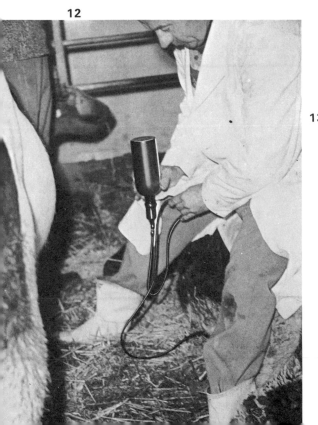

13

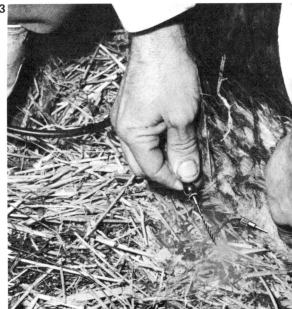

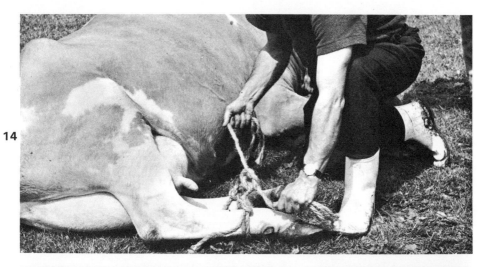

14

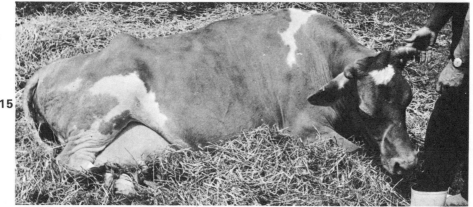

15

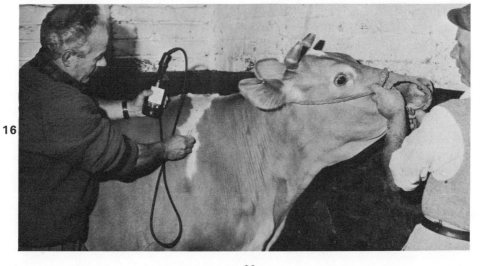

16

SKIN COMPLAINTS

1
Ringworm

ALTHOUGH one of the commonest of all conditions in cattle, ringworm is not, and never should be, a major problem. Nevertheless it is as well to understand it because only by doing so can one keep it in its correct perspective.

Causes
It is caused by several different types of fungi. These fungi wind themselves round the basis of the hairs, making the hairs brittle and loose. At the same time they cause itching which makes the cattle rub themselves on everything. This produces the characteristic rounded bare areas (1).

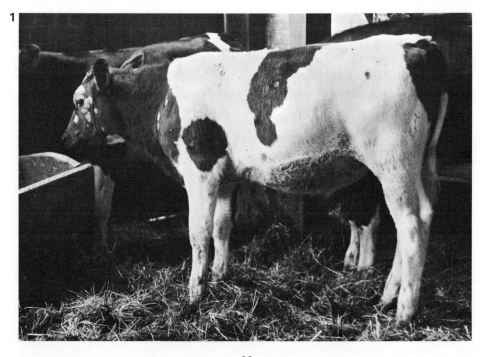

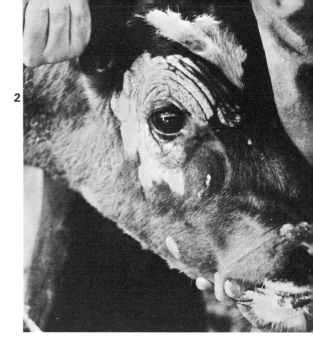

2

Where Fungi Come From

The first and most common source is the 'carrier' cow, stirk or calf, *i.e.,* an animal which shows no symptoms but on which the fungi live and breed. Practically all these carriers are recovered animals—that is, they have had the disease and got better. Recovered human beings can also carry ringworm, and many a herdsman has spread the infection to his calves.

The second source is an infected box in which live fungi can exist for a long time on posts, doors, walls, racks and corn troughs and on the metal of drinking troughs, drinking bowls and stall divisions.

Cause of Flare-up

Ringworm fungi, like all other parasites and germs, grow and thrive best on an underfed animal. Insufficient or bad feeding, therefore, is the greatest contributary cause.

Well-fed animals can, of course, develop ringworm but with them the fungi seldom cause more than the odd lesion. *It is only in the unthrifty calf that ringworm becomes widespread* (2).

How To Recognise It

In the early stages scratching and rubbing are seen but in a very short time the typical round bare patches appear and are soon covered over by a thick horny scab.

It affects chiefly the younger cattle, and the part worst affected is usually the head —especially around the eye and ear.

What To Do

An animal with ringworm develops its own natural resistance after a time. Therefore, if the calves are in reasonably good condition and the ringworms appear in the early spring, then the best practical treatment is to turn the cattle out and forget about them. The ultra-violet rays of the sunlight coupled with the improved nutrition of the grazing will soon help nature to eradicate any average infection.

When the cattle are housed in the winter time the correct procedure in a ringworm outbreak is to provide a full course of 'Fulcin' in the feed (3). Your veterinary surgeon will prescribe the correct dose. After that, the rest should be left to the animal's own natural resistance.

Whatever you do, never repeatedly apply irritant dressings especially the old-fashioned creosote preparations. These damage the hair roots and allow the ringworm to spread more rapidly. They also predispose to secondary bacterial infection and if used around the eyes can cause blindness.

When the fungi become rampant and cover a debilitated calf from head to tail, then the animal should be isolated and treated by a veterinary surgeon. The veterinary surgeon may give intravenous injections of iodine salt solution (4), in addition to the course of 'Fulcin'.

3

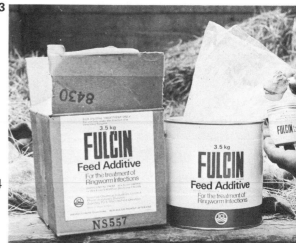

How To Prevent It

Never forget that ringworm thrives on starvation rations. The fungi will never get the better of a well-fed beast. If the growing calves are given good hay, plenty of water and the maximum amounts of high quality protein concentrates (5), then ringworm will never become a serious problem.

Where the odd lesions keep appearing year after year despite the good feeding, the infection is most likely in the calf pen. The thing to do then is to wait until the calves go out to grass and then set to and really clean up the pens. An ordinary rub round with brush and disinfectant is not enough. Get a blowlamp (6) or flame thrower and burn over the walls, stall posts, drinking bowl—the lot—and follow up with a good scrub with hot water and soda. Half measures are no use—make a real thorough job. If you do this, there won't be any fungi in the box for the next batch of calves and the only danger then will be from the odd carrier.

4

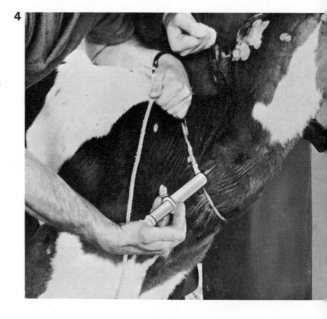

5

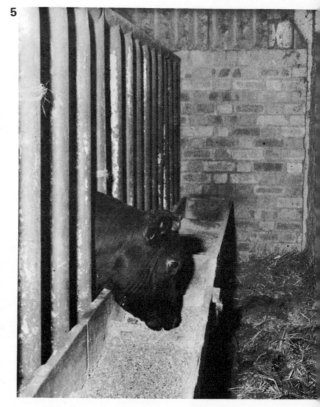

6

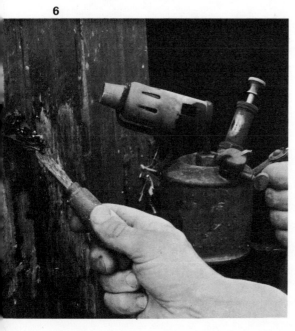

2
Skin Allergy

ALLERGY is the name reserved by medical scientists to describe a condition not fully understood. Skin allergies are among the most difficult of all to fully comprehend or explain, but in the field a practical understanding is all that is necessary.

What Exactly Is An Allergy?
I would describe an allergy simply as an acute reaction between two substances. An acute reaction which manifests itself in many ways—in the case of the skin usually as a painful inflammation of the surface of the teats, udder, belly, and, in severe cases, of the major portion of the body (1).

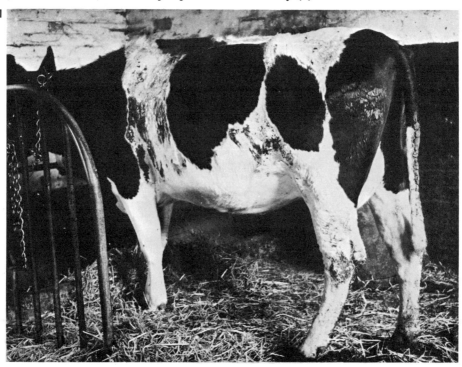

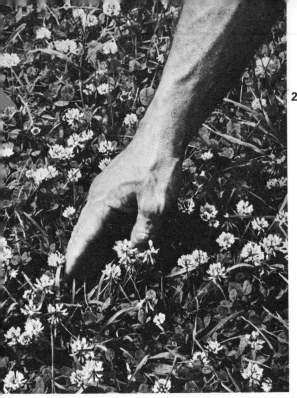

Cause

Occasionally there may be a congenital predisposition but I would say that skin allergies in cattle are mostly protein allergies, that is, some simple protein (technically known as an amino acid) in the hay, concentrates, or most usually in the pasture, when eaten, reacts violently with some similar amino acid already present somewhere in the animal's body.

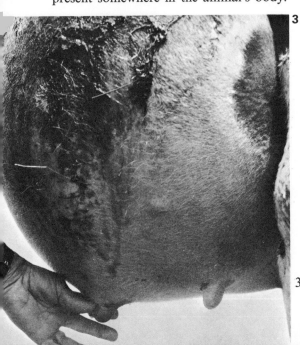

2 This trigger amino acid may be found in certain seasonal weeds or plants but, in my opinion, it is most often found in young clovers (2). I say this because throughout the years most of the cases I have had to treat have been in cattle grazing spring or early summer clover pastures.

Wasp or insect stings are often blamed, and where the white parts of the body are involved, sunlight is alleged by some scientists to be the trigger factor. Stings can and do occasionally cause a transient skin allergy—a reaction which appears suddenly and disappears rapidly—but personally I would question the part played by sunlight, except as a secondary agent after the liver of the affected animal has been damaged during the initial allergy.

How To Recognise the Condition

The first sign of skin allergy is often apparent 'colicy' pains which make the animal kick at her belly, often grunting painfully as she does so.

The skin of the udder teats and underside of the belly becomes hot and painful and the animal will cringe or kick violently when you touch the affected area. Later the affected skin becomes thickened and starts to weep (3).

The surface of the teats and udder often becomes coarse and blue. In advanced **3** severe cases the skin starts to crack and peel off leaving an unholy mess which requires a great deal of nursing (4).

What To Do

It is very important to know exactly what to do at the earliest possible stage in order to prevent a mess or at least save it from spreading to the udder and teats.

The veterinary surgeon should be called immediately. He will confirm the diagnosis and then inject special anti-allergy drugs known as antihistamines (5) or corticosteroids.

He will also immediately dress the udder and the teats with antihistamine or cortisone cream (6). In all cases that I have

37

seen prompt action along these lines has **4**
effectively controlled the condition.

The next essential is a complete change
of diet. If the cow has been at pasture (as
cases usually are) then she should be kept
inside and fed old hay (meadow hay if
possible). The concentrates also should be
changed. I have found that it is best to
feed calf nuts instead of the dairy ration
but only complete change will do.

Can Condition Be Prevented?
Unfortunately, there seems no way of pre-
venting a skin allergy, though fortunately
the condition is usually confined to the
odd one or two animals despite the fact
that the whole herd are ingesting the same **5**
types of protein. Where, as occasionally
happens, several are affected simultaneously then it is wise to change the herd
over to an older, more established pasture.

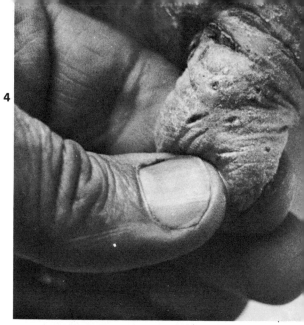

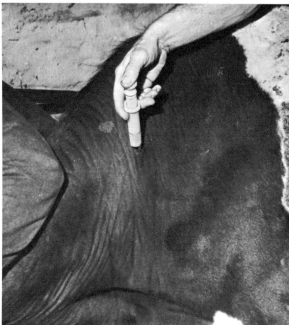

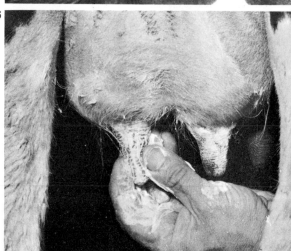

3
Photosensitisation

RECENT work by scientists has shown that hypersensitivity to light, particularly direct sunlight, does indeed occur, though it is relatively uncommon.

What happens is that, under certain circumstances (a few of which are similar to those described under skin allergies), active light rays react with cells in the white or lightly coloured areas of the skin, including the udder and muzzle, and cause inflammation, thickening, and even death of the skin which later peels off to leave sometimes raw infected wounds underneath (1).

Three forms of photosensitisation are now known to occur, the congenital, the primary and the hepatogenous or liver form.

The congenital type occurs only occasionally and susceptible animals show a pink discolouration of the teeth and urine. Such cattle usually lose weight and become anaemic so it is wise to cull them as soon as their weakness is spotted.

Primary photosensitivity is due to the eating, by the cattle, of photosensitising agents contained in certain plants, weeds, clovers and rape.

Liver photosensitisation occurs when the liver cells are damaged and are therefore unable to destroy photosensitising agents absorbed from the digestive tract—agents like certain breakdown products of chlorophyll, the green pigment of plants.

Treatment
House the affected animal in a dark box for at least a week and have her injected daily, with cortisone preparations, by your veterinary surgeon. He will no doubt prescribe a suitable local dressing for the damaged skin.

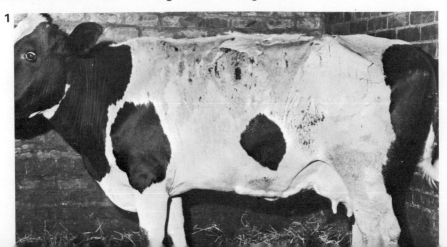

1

4
Warts

WARTS in human beings and in animals very often disappear almost spectacularly. The explanation of this phenomenon is that the body acquires a strong natural resistance.

Cause

There now seems little doubt that warts are caused by a virus infection. Formerly they were regarded as parasitic growths of unknown origin, but now virologists have proved that they can be transmitted to laboratory and other animals.

Looking back over the years I can recall abundant evidence to back up the virologists' findings. Warts of all shapes and sizes have occurred in horses, donkeys, cattle, sheep, pigs, dogs, cats and even in the odd monkey or two (1—wart or angleberry removed from a pony).

I have seen the briskets of heifers and bullocks so heavily laden that walking was an effort and then quite suddenly, often whilst awaiting surgical removal, the warts have died and dropped off (2).

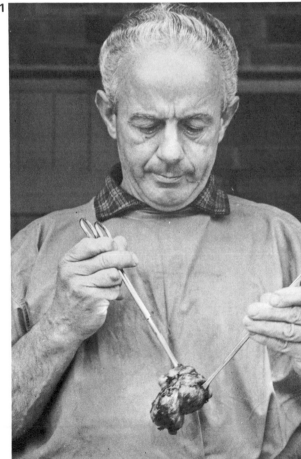

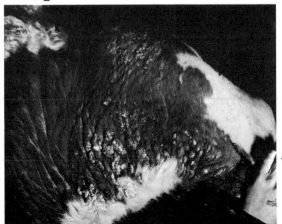

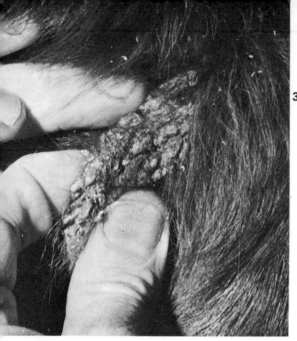

I have seen unsightly ulcerating angleberries on a horse disappear like magic after a summer at grass. In fact, in all but the worst affected, time seems to be the main curative agent.

One thing I have noticed though is that the really severe wart invasions occur in animals in low condition. This, of course, bears out the general undisputed fact that poor condition and lowered resistance are predisposing causes of all bacterial, viral or fungal invasions.

Some of you might say that this doesn't always follow in relation to 'warty teats' which are often seen on heifers and cows in top-class condition. In such cases the explanation is that the virus is a powerful one and the affected animals are being attacked for the first time and have not yet had sufficient time to acquire an immunity.

Symptoms
The warts just appear and seem to grow and spread rapidly. As with practically all other diseases, antibodies start appearing in the bloodstream 14 days after the original wart infection but thereafter in the case of the warts, the antibodies have a long hard uphill fight to control and defeat the invasion. Almost invariably,

3 therefore, the warts manifest themselves clearly.

Occasionally the warts become malignant, but this only happens when cancerous cells start to grow in the damaged tissue. For the most part they are benign and can be cured. The wart illustrated (3) was benign but had to be cut out because the farmer hadn't the patience to wait for it to drop off.

Prevention
The obvious golden rule in prevention is to keep the young cattle well fed and in good growing condition—warts, like lice, mange and ringworm, thrive and play havoc among the undernourished stores.

Apart from this simple 'must', there is little else to be done although in any particularly severe outbreak it is possible to inoculate with an 'autogenous' vaccine, which is a vaccine prepared from a sample of the warts prevailing (4).

It is important that the vaccine should be made from the particular warts on a farm because undoubtedly there are many different strains of wart virus and a vaccine prepared against warts in the South of England would be unlikely to afford any protection against the warts of the Midlands or North and vice versa.

Just one important point—once a heifer

4

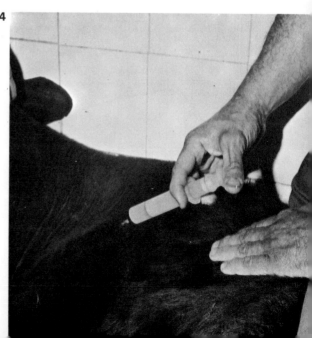

has overcome a wart infection she retains
a powerful natural resistance. It would,
therefore, be unwise and unnecessary to
sell her in the fear of recurrence.

Treatment
Treatment depends largely on extent and
site of lesions and your veterinary surgeon
should be left to decide and prescribe. If
the warts are on the body and not too
extensive he will probably advise leaving
them alone and concentrating on main-
taining the animal in good condition.
Local applications of caustic are dangerous
and ineffective. Glacial acetic acid has
been widely recommended and used on
teats, but I have found it irritant and
inconsistent.

In gross infestations the removal of even
part of the mass is often sufficient to
enable the body resistance to take over
and complete the cure.

But it is with warty teats (5) that perhaps the most persistent economic trouble
arises and here there are one or two
sensible practical hints for the herd-owner.

Practical Hints
In a dry heifer or cow, particularly in the
summer, it is unwise to attempt to pull off
all the warts (6) because extensive wounds
will be left on the teats and mastitis will
be a near certainty.

If, however, the affected animal can be
handled regularly I think it is a good idea
for the stockman to pull off one small
wart every other day provided he dis-
infects his hands thoroughly before doing
so and massages a small quantity of
sulphanilamide into the wound immediately afterwards (7). If, of course, only
one wart is present this should be done as
soon as it is spotted.

An extremely useful daily dressing is the
old-fashioned 'salicylic ointment'. This can
easily be had on prescription from your
veterinary surgeon and should be massaged
gently into the warty mass once daily (8).

Almost any antiseptic application is a
safe line of treatment for warty teats

5

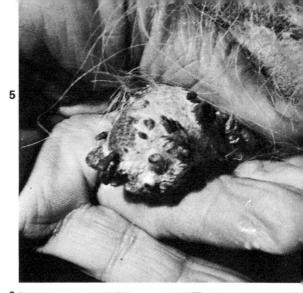

6

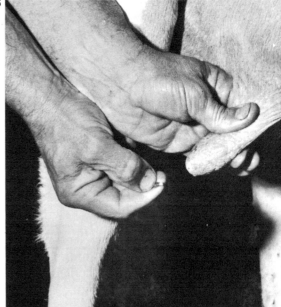

7

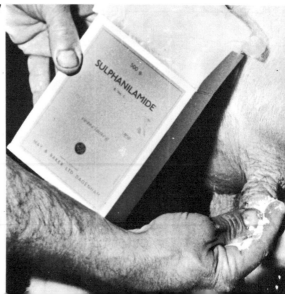

42

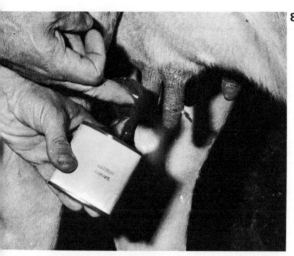

8

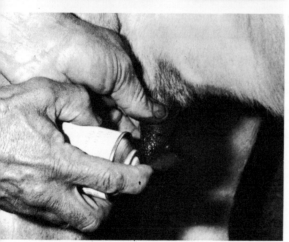

9

provided the antiseptic is not too irritant. Many of the modern aerosols are ideal for this purpose (9).

One last word: don't be tempted to resort to the primitive method of applying ligatures around the wart bases. Rubber bands, cotton and silk threads, *etc.,* merely produce ulcerating wounds which cry out for invasion by mastitis, tetanus and other germs.

EYE DISORDERS

1
Chaff in Eye

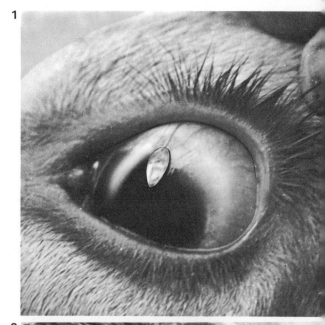

ONE of the trickiest jobs a stockman has to do is to deal with chaff in a cow's eye (1). There are many so-called traditional remedies like blowing sugar into the eye, inserting castor oil, or attempting to flick the chaff away with the corner of a handkerchief.

Here, however, is a simple method of getting chaff out.

Take any tube of eye ointment—it has to be ointment and not an oily suspension. Squeeze a small quantity out on to the end of the nozzle, sufficient to form a sticky pad (2).

Very slowly, so as not to alarm the animal, move the padded nozzle towards the eye. Then when a little way from the eye deftly press the pad against the chaff. The cow will involuntarily pull its head away, and the chaff will be left sticking to the ointment (3).

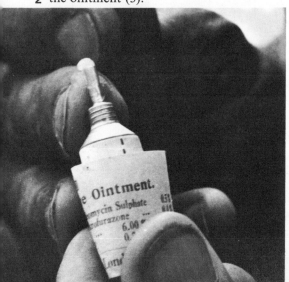

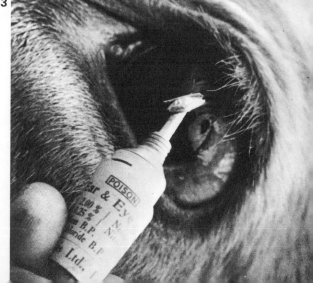

It's a good idea to insert a small 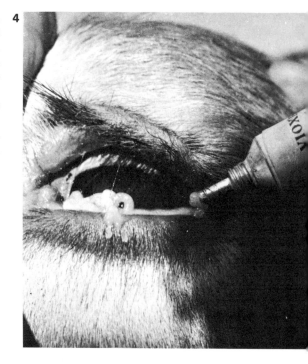 quantity of the eye ointment along the lower lid when the chaff has been removed. (4). This will combat any infection. A good eye ointment obtained from your veterinary surgeon produces very little irritation. Within 24 hours or less the eye should be back to normal.

Don't keep bodging— if you don't succeed in two or three attempts, send for your veterinary surgeon. He will probably spray the surface of the eye with a local anaesthetic solution and pick the chaff off with a pair of forceps.

2
New Forest Disease
(Infectious Keratitis)

NEW FOREST DISEASE (1) affects the eyes of cattle of all ages, expecially year-lings and calves.

1

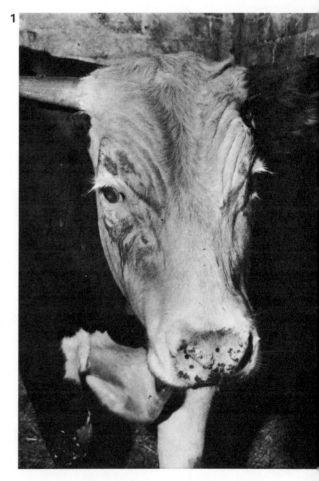

Cause
It is caused by a germ called the *Moraxella bovis.*

Where Germ Comes From
Although not, so far, scientifically proved, the bug apparently lurks in the eyes of many normal animals and becomes active only when there is some damage to the eye surface—damage caused by foreign matter (2) such as dust particles, chaff, irritation by flies, *etc.* This fact probably explains why the disease is most common in the summer, and often flares up during dry, windy weather.

2

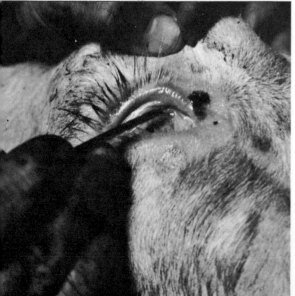

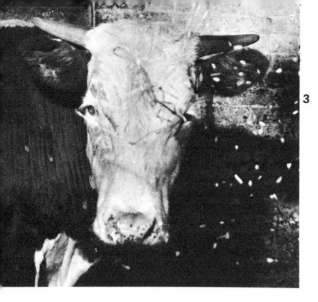

3

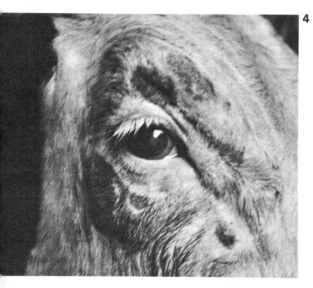

4

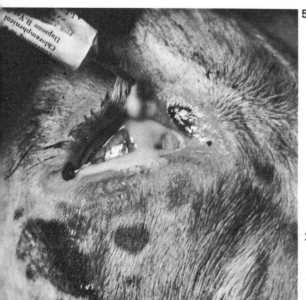

5

The dust or chaff (3), which can fly about in a loose box or open yard, produces an irritation which allows the resident germ to get going. The *Moraxella* pierces the surface of the centre part of the eye (called the cornea) and starts to multiply.

If untreated, it forms first of all a white pin-head which rapidly increases in size.

If still untreated, a yellow pointing abscess may form which eventually ruptures, leaving a filthy raw ulcer which may take up to three months to heal.

During this time the germ in its most powerful form is present in all the eye discharge. The wind may blow such discharge over considerable distances. This probably explains why the disease spreads often alarmingly in a herd.

The earliest symptom is a running eye (4) or a closed eye. Both eyes may be affected. Because of its rapid development and spread it is very important to treat the disease at the earliest possible stage. Once the condition has been diagnosed on your farm, therefore, you should be on the constant look-out for the 'streaming eye'.

How To Treat Condition

There are a number of first-class preparations available in the form of ointment, emulsions or drops. I have personally found that the most successful application is an emulsion containing chloramphenicol and cortesone. A single application inserted early on will often effect a cure within a few hours. Even after the eye is 'marked', results can be quite spectacular but the eye may have to be dressed twice daily for a considerable time (5).

Unfortunately, New Forest disease cannot be prevented, but it can be controlled by a constant vigil and prompt treatment.

MOUTH AILMENTS

1
Wooden Tongue
(Actinobacillosis)

TWO organisms are concerned:
- (a) A germ called the *Actinobacillus lignieresi.*
- (b) A fungus called the *Streptothrix actinomyces* or *actinomyces bovis:* this fungus is more often known as the Ray Fungus.

Where the Germ and Fungi Come From
Both the fungus and the germ are normal residents of the mouth, lying dormant in the tonsils chiefly. They can also be present in lymph glands in other parts of the body.

What Triggers Off Disease
When any of the soft tissues of the mouth, *e.g.,* the tongue, lips, soft palate or cheeks, are scratched or cut (1) the fungus or germ may take the chance to multiply and grow in the damaged tissues.

Exactly the same thing can happen when there is a wound in the lining of the pharynx, larynx, oesophagus or the first and second stomachs, that is, the rumen and reticulum. The reticulum or second stomach is particularly prone to 'wooden tongue' because there portions of wire or nails and other foreign bodies are trapped and these are constantly liable to scratch the lining. Where these soft tissues of the digestive tract are involved (2) the germ —the *Actinobacillus lignieresi*—is nearly always at fault.

If the ray fungus gains entrance into a

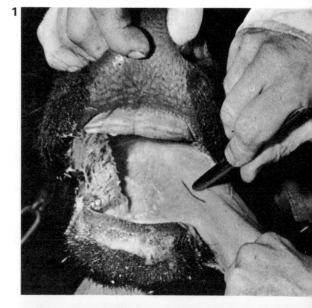

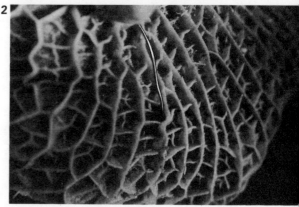

bone cavity, as, for example, when heifers
and bullocks are shedding teeth, it can
cause infection and swelling of the jaw
bone (3). This actinomyces of the bone is
a very much more serious condition than
infection of the soft tissue.

Less frequently a wooden tongue infection can flare up in the liver, lungs or
udder. Where the bone or udder is affected
the Ray Fungus is usually the culprit.

What Happens
When they multiply, both the germs and
fungi produce faci of pus which surround
themselves with hard fibrous tissue (4).
This causes the hard 'wooden' feeling.

Symptoms
When the cow's tongue becomes 'wooden',
grazing and eating become well-nigh impossible and naturally the animal slobbers
at the mouth (5) and sinks rapidly in
condition. Usually the glands under the
jaw become hard and swollen also.

Stomach infection is difficult to diagnose,
the only signs being a capricious appetite
and a slowly progressive loss in condition
in otherwise healthy cattle.

Chance of Recovery
When the bone is affected the prospects
of recovery are nil, but nearly all soft tissue
infections respond extremely well to treatment. It is wise to leave the diagnosis and
treatment to your veterinary surgeon
because occasionally identical symptoms
can be produced by other factors.

Your veterinary surgeon will treat the
condition by injecting either antibiotics,
sulpha drugs or iodine preparations, depending on the lesions.

Prevention
A practical prevention, as yet widely used
only in South America, is the daily feeding
of small quantities of iodine. Iodine has
a curative effect on wooden tongue and
apparently small quantities such as are
present in the average iodised mineral do
exert considerable control.

3

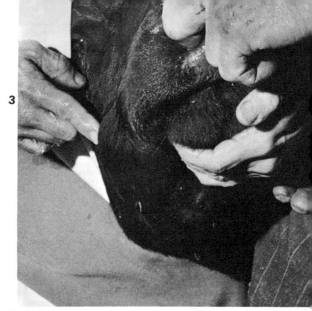

4

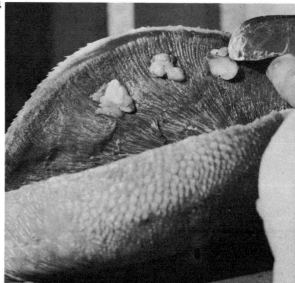

5

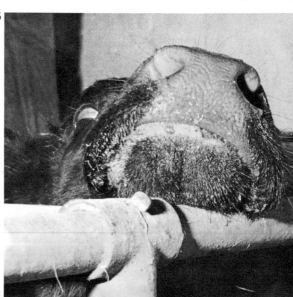

2
Foot and Mouth Disease

WHENEVER there is a slobbering bovine, of course, the possibility of foot and mouth disease must never be overlooked.

Cause
A virus. There are several types of virus and a number of strains of each type. Where does the virus come from? Chiefly imported meat. It can live in frozen meat and especially in the bone marrow for a very long time.

Symptoms
In the dairy herd or in housed feeding cattle, unmistakable general signs are usually rapidly apparent—a sudden drop in the herd gallonage and the appearance, in a very short time, of other cattle similarly affected.

The individually affected animals, apart from slobbering, sucking and showing characteristic blisters in their mouths (1), run a high fever and very soon exhibit obvious pain and discomfort when standing (2) or attempting to walk. If the cow lives long enough the teats become involved (3). In calves, deaths may occur.

1

2
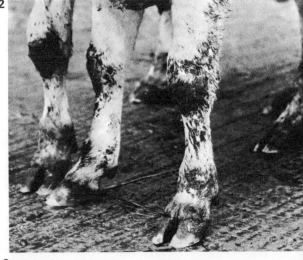

3
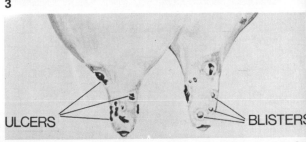

ULCERS   BLISTERS

With outlying cattle, the evidence is not so apparent, but any lame slobbering animal should be reported to the police or to a veterinary surgeon immediately. During a foot and mouth outbreak, the entire country is alerted and it is the duty of every stockowner to be extra vigilant and observant. The slightest suspicion must be reported at once.

Prevention

In Great Britain foot and mouth disease is controlled by a slaughter policy. The question is often asked, particularly by laymen, why not vaccinate? There are several reasons. Apart altogether from the expense and difficulty in handling hill sheep, especially, a vaccine prepared against a particular strain of one type of virus gives no protection against the other strains or against the other types. Also there is a danger that a vaccinated animal may remain a 'carrier' and this possibility could ruin our export trade. The vaccine cannot be used in young calves, which are the most vulnerable of all livestock, and it is also unsatisfactory in sheep and pigs. Without a doubt, the slaughter policy is much more satisfactory in every way.

3
Mucosal Disease

ANOTHER disease of cattle which can produce slobbering and stiffness is the condition called mucosal disease. This is most usually seen in feeding cattle, though it can and does affect cows and I have seen it in a group of calves.

Cause
A virus in some respects similar to the foot and mouth viruses, though it is nothing like as acutely contagious. Again and again I have seen mucosal disease affecting only one of a large group of cattle. Often there is no apparent reason for the flare up, though sometimes it can be attributed to the stress of a long journey or to rapid changes in atmospheric temperature and conditions.

Symptoms
In the early stages—a high temperature up to 106°F with reddening of the lining of the mouth and nostrils and complete inappetence. This stage may last for only 48 hours or less and is often missed, especially among feeding cattle.

Secondary to the virus attack, bacteria move in and cause a stinking discharge from the mouth and nostrils (1): and ulcers in the mouth and nostrils, and occasionally feet ulcers not unlike those of foot and mouth. Because of the bowel damage there is usually a foul smelling diarrhoea (2) and an acute pneumonia may develop. The bacterial invasion usually shoots the temperature up again.

1

2

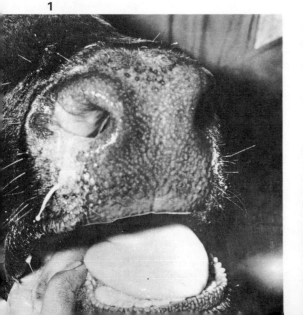
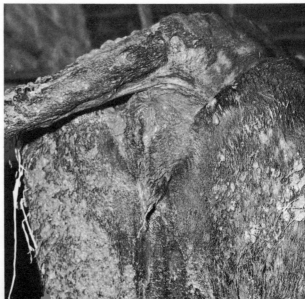

Treatment

Obviously, diagnosis and treatment is very much a matter for your veterinary surgeon. I have found that acute cases are seldom worth treating and, if the temperature is normal or subnormal I never hesitate to have the animal slaughtered for salvage. It is my experience that such cases kill out very well, no doubt because of the dehydration caused by the diarrhoea and because the virus damage is usually confined to the lining of the digestive tract.

Medicinal treatment comprises sulpha drugs and antibiotics given both by injection and by the mouth. A protracted course is usually required. In my opinion it is uneconomical and unwise to treat any save the mild cases of mucosal disease.

Prevention

There is no vaccine against mucosal and no reliable routine preventative husbandry measures.

LUNG TROUBLES

1

Husk

(Parasitic Bronchitis)

HUSK is caused by a group of lung worms called the *Dictyocauli*.

How Worms Produce Their Effect

Inside the lungs of an infected animal or a 'carrier' animal, there are male and female worms (1). Copulation takes place and a single female worm may lay several thousand eggs per day. Each egg contains an immature but potential adult male or female worm.

The eggs are coughed up from the lungs into the mouth. They are swallowed and passed down through the stomach and intestines. During the journey they change into what we call first-stage larvae.

These larvae are passed out with the dung on to the pastures. In the warm damp conditions that prevail close to the dung pat the larvae undergo two changes in less than a week to become 'infective'.

When the unsuspecting calf eats the contaminated grass, the infective larvae pass down into the small intestine. There they bore through the wall of the intestine and migrate through the body until they reach the lungs, where they move into the larger air spaces. Here, approximately 28 days after being eaten, they grow into adult male and female worms ready to start breeding many thousands more of their kind.

The infective larvae in ideal conditions of shade, warmth and moisture can live on the pasture for over 12 months, though if there is a hot dry summer or a very cold

1

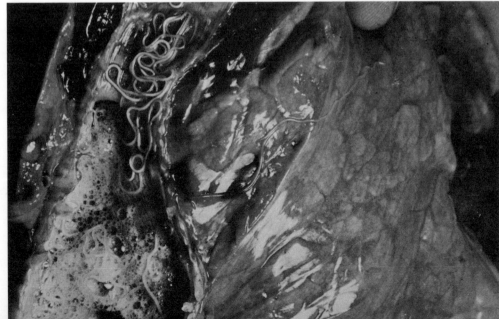

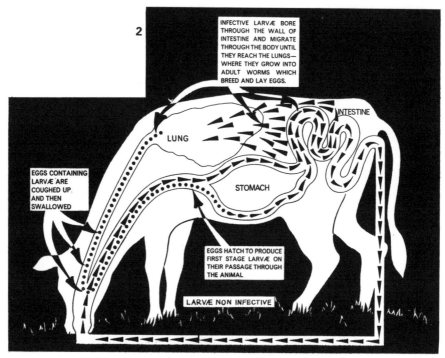

2

INFECTIVE LARVÆ BORE THROUGH THE WALL OF INTESTINE AND MIGRATE THROUGH THE BODY UNTIL THEY REACH THE LUNGS— WHERE THEY GROW INTO ADULT WORMS WHICH BREED AND LAY EGGS.

INTESTINE

LUNG

EGGS CONTAINING LARVÆ ARE COUGHED UP. AND THEN SWALLOWED

STOMACH

EGGS HATCH TO PRODUCE FIRST STAGE LARVÆ ON THEIR PASSAGE THROUGH THE ANIMAL

LARVÆ NON INFECTIVE

FIRST-STAGE LARVÆ FROM DUNG OF INFECTED
ANIMALS DEVELOP IN ABOUT SEVEN DAYS TO
THE INFECTIVE STAGE.

winter, their period of survival may be cut down to less than a month. During the heat of the day they go down into the base of the grass for protection, but in the mornings and evenings they crawl up the blades of grass ready to be picked up (2).

One other method of spread is by a fungus called the *Pilobolus*. This fungus grows out from the dung pats. The fungus carries the infective larvae in its top portion. After a time the top portion bursts and the larvae are blown $6\frac{1}{2}'$ in the air and up to 10' all around (3).

It is not difficult to understand how a

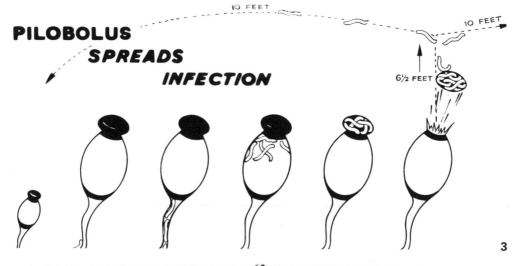

10 FEET

PILOBOLUS
SPREADS
INFECTION

10 FEET

6½ FEET

3

few infected calves, each with a large number of adult worms in the lungs and each female worm laying thousands of eggs per day, can soon contaminate many acres of land. In fact, in three weeks, one calf can pass enough larvae to infect 3,000 other calves.

As you can well understand, a few thousand larvae penetrating into a lung can soon play havoc. They do, in fact, cause a pneumonia, but the damage caused by the larvae often allows germs to get in also and the germs cause a severe and often fatal bacterial pneumonia (4).

How To Recognise Husk
Though coughing is often the first alarm sign that registers, the earliest danger sign in husk is the increased rate of respiration. In the beginning the calf may breathe at

terised by a desperate grunting or gasping for breath (5).

What To Do
It is essential that a veterinary surgeon should confirm the diagnosis before prescribing treatment because it is possible to confuse husk with a virus pneumonia (often called 'cuffing' pneumonia). If the veterinary surgeon has any doubt, he will examine faeces samples before starting treatment.

There is now widely available a specific curative drug called 'Diethylcarbamezine'. Diethylcarbamezine (6) should be injected intramuscularly once daily for three days. Treatment will be highly successful provided it is started as soon as the coughing is heard. Treatment has to be combined with practical husbandry precautions.

4

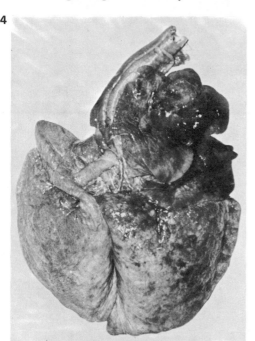

5

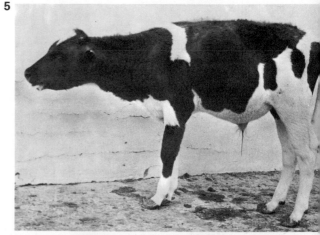

6

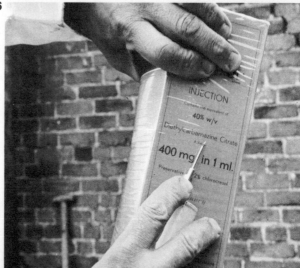

twice the normal rate before it starts to cough. When the coughing does start it is accentuated when the calf is chased round.

As the condition gets worse, the calves rapidly lose condition and many of them may develop a fatal pneumonia charac-

How To Prevent Husk

The oral vaccine now available against husk (comprising live larvae weakened by X-rays) is one of the best vaccines ever discovered (7), but its use has to be combined with commonsense husbandry.

It is important to remember that the dangerous carriers of husk are the two-year-olds, *i.e.,* animals which have had husk the year before, have apparently recovered, but which still harbour the worms in their lungs.

Obviously, therefore, the newly-turned-out vaccinated calves should never be turned out to graze with or after the two-year-olds. If possible, they should be turned on to a pasture which has been rested com-pletely throughout the winter, and once there they should be kept there. Such a pasture, if infected, will only be lightly infected and the vaccinated calves will pick up additional small doses of larvae which will reinforce the immunity given by the oral vaccine.

One other very important preventive hint. Wherever you have husk, you also have stomach and bowel worms. The grazing calves should, therefore, be dosed for ordinary worms at least twice during their grazing season, the first dose to be given six weeks after the calves have been turned out (8). The husk vaccine gives no protection against stomach and bowel worms.

7

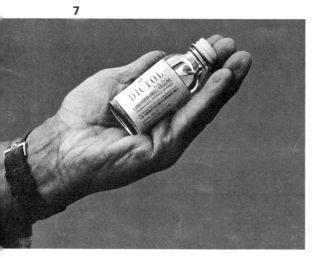

8

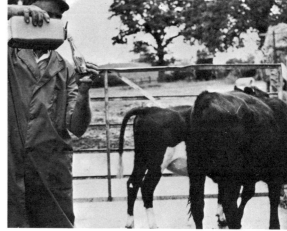

2
Virus Pneumonia

VIRUS PNEUMONIA in cattle (sometimes called cuffing pneumonia) costs the farming industry hundreds of thousands of pounds each year.

Type of Animal Usually Attacked
Younger calves are the more susceptible (1), though I have seen it in animals up to 18 months old and just occasionally in adult cattle.

Symptoms
The first symptom is a persistent dry cough. In fact, coughing, which is due to bronchitis, can be present for some time before the pneumonia sets in. When the pneumonia starts the calf goes off its food, runs a temperature of about 106° (2) and breathes heavily. If untreated it starts to grunt and behave exactly like a calf with acute parasitic pneumonia (husk).

Eight viruses are now known to be associated with calf pneumonia. They are:

Parainfluenza 3, Bovine Adenovirus 1, Bovine Adenovirus 2, Bovine Adenovirus 3, Infectuous Bovine Rhinotracheitis, Mucosal Disease Virus, Bovine Reoviruses, Bedsonia Organisms.

An impressive list—but the majority of cases involve only the *Parainfluenza 3,* the *Adenovirus 3,* or the *Bedsonia Organisms*: and it is against these three that

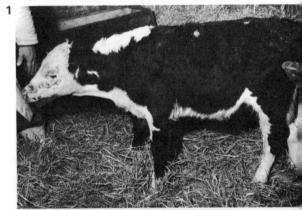

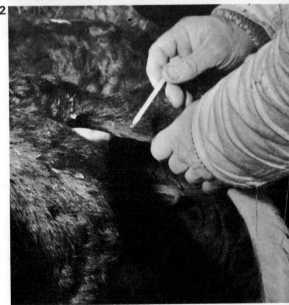

vaccinal research has so far been concentrated. The viruses cause an initial bronchitis which lowers the resistance of the lung and allows secondary bacteria to set up the pneumonia (3).

Where Viruses Come From

Like all bugs they live and persist in carrier animals; that is, animals which have recovered from a mild attack and continue to carry the virus without showing any symptoms. The viruses live usually in the tonsils at the back of the throat (4). Most adult cattle probably carry the viruses in the same way as most humans carry the virus of the common cold. The adults carry a powerful natural immunity but often remain dangerous carriers.

The answers?—The viruses come usually from bought-in calves that have been infected either in intensive houses, at markets, or from recovered 'carriers'. The

What Causes Virus To Flare Up?

Once again it is the old story of lowered resistance—bad management and poor feeding, but most of all bad housing. The pneumonia viruses seem to thrive best in calves which are exposed to draughts (5–6)—exactly the same story as with the common cold virus in humans.

Another factor, almost as lethal, is an atmosphere which is subjected to extremes of temperature. Such an atmosphere is often to be found in a building with an uninsulated galvanised roof (7). Invariably such buildings are too hot in the summer and excessively cold in the winter; or moderately warm during the day and extremely cold during the night.

Another possible, though less frequent cause, is an under-populated building; that is, a large box with a high roof containing only a few calves (8). Such calves are not sufficiently dense to warm up the

3

4

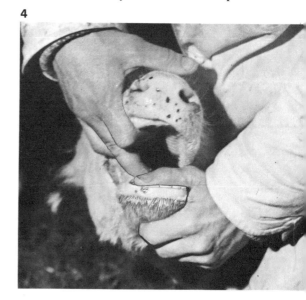

viruses live only for a short time outside the animals, so that any building that has been completely emptied of stock should be clear comparatively quickly, especially if the buildings have been thoroughly cleaned out.

available air and to maintain it at a constant temperature.

The final resistance lowering factor is the fog of excessive condensation; that is, a wet fog produced by hot air condensing against the cold roof (9). I have found that this factor will help only to perpetuate or

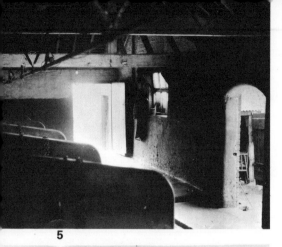

5

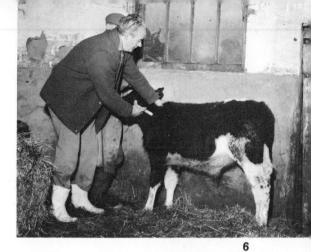

6

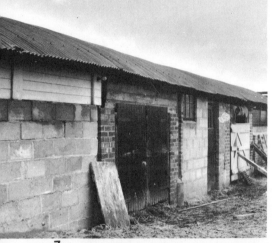

7

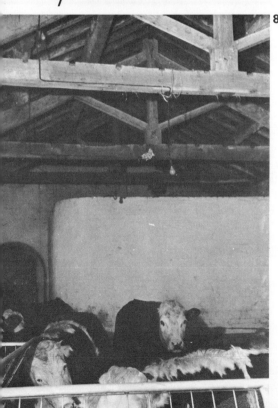

8

spread a strong active infection. It is unlikely to trigger off the initial attack; certainly much less likely to do so than draughts. Bad drainage in a pen will also contribute to excess condensation.

Treatment
Fortunately, provided the case is taken in time, the secondary pneumonia can be cured by most of the modern antibiotics, though some of the secondary bacteria, particularly a germ called the *Pasteurella,* require a powerful drug blitz. Treatment should be continued for at least five days after the calf's temperature has returned to normal (10).

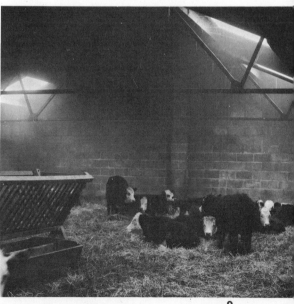

9

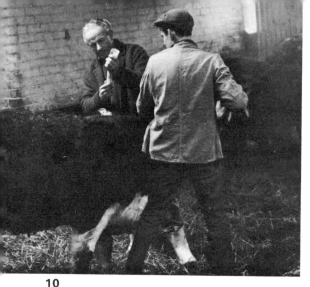

10

Prevention Management and Control

Virus pneumonia can be controlled to some extent by commonsense housing. In fact, one of the worst outbreaks ever which occurred a few years ago in the north of England was completely eliminated by doing nothing apart from altering and correcting the house.

The ideal to aim at is the provision of a draught-proof kennel for the calves to live in. This can be done in any shed or box by providing a false roof of wire netting and straw or slats and sacks, or any other available scrap material. *But, and this is the important point, it must be absolutely draught-proof—the false roof should fit tightly against three solid walls and only the front part of the kennel should be open.* All cracks and crevices in the three walls should be effectively filled in (11).

11

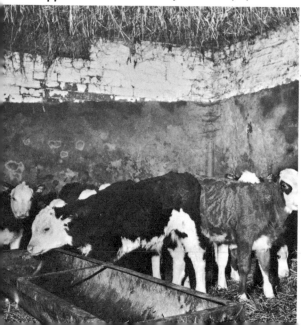

Wire netting and straw make perhaps the best improvisation and cost little or nothing, but any old waste material will do. Galvanised sheets can be used for the false roof provided they are covered by a good coating of sacks or straw.

Any farm building, no matter how old or dilapidated, can be made comparatively safe for calves in this simple way.

Getting Rid of Virus from a Shed

The only way to clean up a box or shed is to empty the building of all stock, clean it down (12), scrub it out with hot water, soda and antiseptic and leave it empty for 14 days. The box or building must be completely empty. If you leave one calf stirk or cow within that building or inside a communicating box, then the virus will reside and persist within that animal and will spread to any calves brought in subsequently.

Prevention By Vaccination

There is available a new vaccine which protects against the three main viruses mentioned earlier: *Parainfluenza 3*, *Adenovirus 3* and *Bedsonia*. What I like about it is that it can be used at any age from two weeks onwards. The dose is just 2 ccs, and it is injected underneath the skin about half-way up the side of the neck (13).

A second dose is given one month later and that's it—no further booster doses are required. You may get a slight swelling at the site of injection but this usually disappears in a few weeks.

But just a few words of warning!— Never vaccinate unhealthy sickly calves and don't whatever you do get the idea that the vaccine is going to take the place of good management and good housing— it *won't*. The vaccine's true potential will only be realised if the calves are housed in a reasonable environment.

The avoidance of draughts, overcrowding, and poor ventilation are just as vital with vaccinated as with non-vaccinated calves—Why?—because no vaccine can be expected to stand up against the stresses

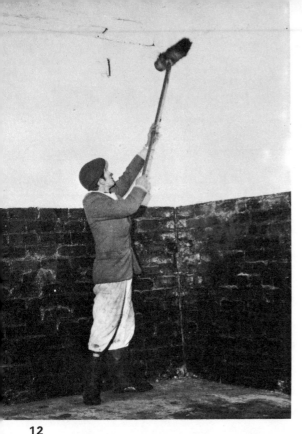

12

of extremes of temperature or of lack of air.

I think and I have written and said this on many occasions—that it is comparatively easy to get a satisfactory environment for growing calves by inexpensive improvisation even in the worst of bad buildings.

13

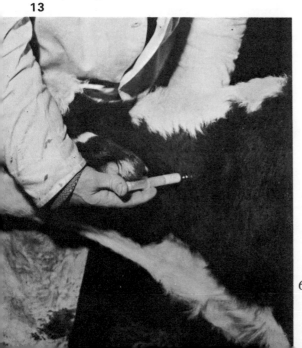

Let me just repeat for emphasis—you can eliminate draught simply by creating a kennel or kennels within the main building, always remembering that the kennel must be completely closed above and on three sides and that the kennel roof must not be too high. You can insulate any calf pen by lining it with straw bales and you can make the false roof with wire netting and straw.

You can avoid excess humidity by making sure the pens are drained properly.

You can get rid of the stale air simply by having an inlet for fresh air which will guard against direct draught and an outlet at the highest point or in an opposite corner of the main building. The stale air will rise to the top of the kennels but will filter out at a steady pace if there is a free movement of air above. A good percentage of the cooler fresh air will gravitate quietly into the kennels and keep the atmosphere clear.

But obviously each farm has its own particular problems to overcome and my advice is to consult both your veterinary surgeon and your NAAS officer together. Ask your vet to bring the buildings officer or vice versa—both will break their necks to co-operate and only good will result.

STOMACH TROUBLES

1
Bloat

THERE are two types of bloat—ordinary bloat and frothy bloat. Both occur when the cow's first stomach or rumen fills up with gases (1).

In the ordinary type of bloat the gases, which are formed during the breakdown of the foodstuffs by bacteria, accumulate in the upper part of the first stomach.

Although serious enough in itself, ordinary bloat is not usually fatal, since the free gas in the upper part of the stomach is usually regurgitated when the cow is exercised or drenched.

By far the more serious type of bloat, and the one which we mostly have to contend with especially at turning-out time, is the frothy type.

In frothy bloat the rapidly forming gases, instead of passing freely to the top of the stomach, are trapped among the ruminal contents in the form of minute bubbles of froth (2).

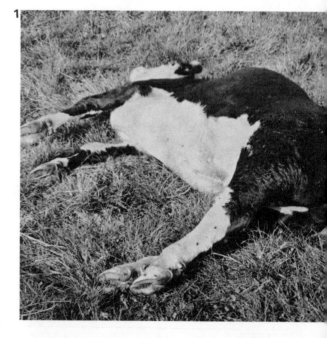

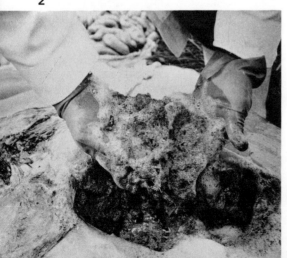

This trapping occurs when the ruminal contents are thick, tacky and tenacious. They are like this when the salivary glands which open into the cow's mouth do not produce enough saliva to mix with the foodstuffs as they are chewed and swallowed.

It is believed that the action of the salivary glands is stimulated, not only by chewing, but also by the amount of coarse fibre in the cow's second stomach or reticulum (3).

73

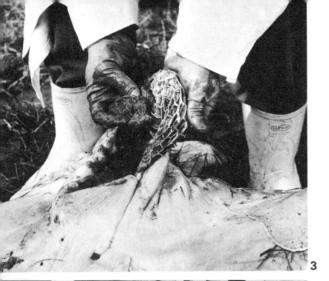

3

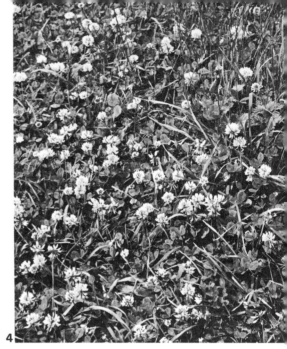

4

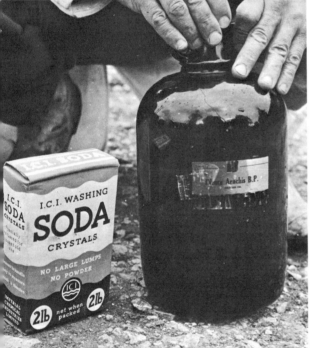

5

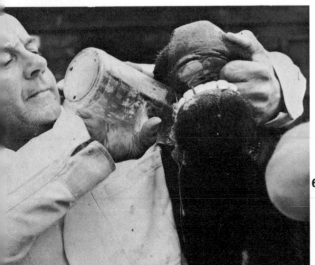

6

It is quite obvious, therefore, that frothy bloat is liable to occur whenever there is a deficiency of fibre in the diet. This means that the most dangerous pastures are the short rapidly growing clovers with little length of fibrous stem.

Pastures with some length are much safer and in general the longer the grasses the safer they are (4).

What To Do

First of all, if the cow is on pasture and if she can stand and walk, bring her into the farmyard immediately.

The best two first-aid remedies for bloat are *Oleum Arachis* (commonly known as peanut oil) or ordinary washing soda crystals (5).

The doses are either a pint of peanut oil in some warm water or $\frac{1}{4}$ lb. of washing soda dissolved in hot water and diluted to approximately one pint with cold.

Now the drenching. Be careful with bloat cases. Don't hold the nose; pass the arm over the top of the nose and insert the hand into the mouth, as in the picture (6). Take your time, and don't try to pour the whole bottle over at once. Several times cows have recovered from bloat but subsequently died because some of the drench went into the lungs through over-haste.

After the drenching, halter the cow and make her walk around the yard. Have a feel on the left flank fairly frequently to make sure it is not too tightly blown (7).

If the bloat is rapidly getting worse in spite of the drench and there is still no sign of your vet, it may be a matter for emergency puncture. The correct site is this fairly wide circle on the left flank, equidistant from the last rib, the point of the hip, and the bottom of the spine (8).

If you have time, shave the centre of the target area with a razor blade or scalpel, swab with antiseptic and cut through the skin, once again using the razor blade or scalpel. The size of the cut should be $\frac{1}{2}''$ to $1''$ (9).

Now the puncturing instrument (10). The trocar and cannula is best, and on farms where bloat is a problem it is advisable that one should be on hand. Push the trocar and cannula straight in as far as it will go—you won't harm the cow and you won't do any permanent damage.

Now remove the trocar, holding the cannula in position with the finger while doing so. This leaves the far end of the cannula inside the rumen. In the majority of cases the relief is very rapid. It is best

7

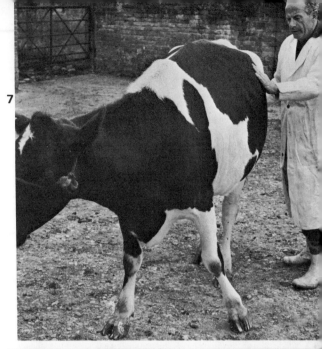

8

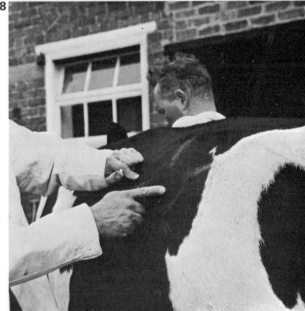

9

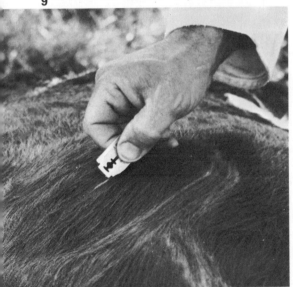

10

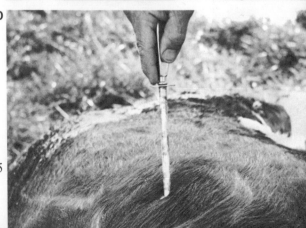

75

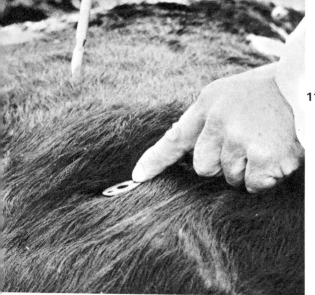

11 to hold the cannula in position until the veterinary surgeon arrives (11).

If you have no trocar, a bread knife, or a butcher's knife like this one, will do. Be bold. Stick the knife in right to the hilt, then partially withdraw it and turn the blade in a full circle (12). Once more the gas will bubble forth and relief will be rapid. Don't forget! A bold incision in the left flank equidistant from the last rib, the point of the hip, and the bottom of the spine. Suffer from timidity or apprehension and you'll finish up with a dead cow. *Just one word of warning, never under any circumstances puncture a cow on the*
12 *right side—always in the left flank.*

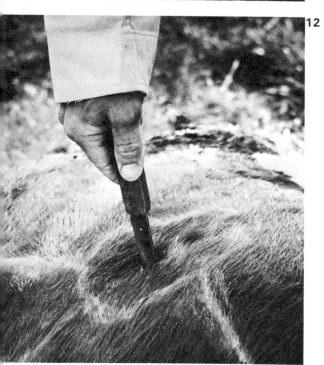

How To Prevent Bloat

1. Before turning on to the dangerous type of young lush pastures, particularly if there is a clover dominance in that pasture, all animals should be given some fibre in the form of hay or straw (13). Alternatively, the area of pasture to be grazed should be sprinkled over with the hay or straw.
2. The grazing should be controlled by paddocks, using the electric fence or by allowing only short periods of eating time —preferably both.
3. If available, farmyard manure should be distributed on the pastures during the winter time, and a correct pasture balance should be established between clovers and other grasses. *Clover dominance is always dangerous.*

13

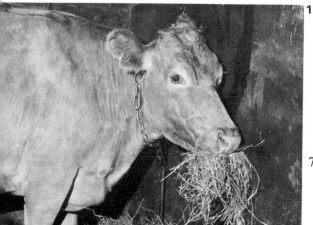

76

2
Recurrent Bloat

RECURRENT BLOAT is simply a condition when calves, cows or steers blow up more than once within a comparatively short time.

Cause

The condition can be due to any one of four things:

The first and most common cause is an enlargement of one or more of the lymphatic glands which lie on each side of the oesophagus (food pipe) inside the chest. The enlargement is due to an infection of these glands, and the pressure exerted on the oesophagus by the swollen gland prevents the regurgitation of gas from the stomach. In my experience the most common germ involved in these glandular enlargements is the wooden tongue germ, *viz*. the *Actinobacillus lignier-*

esi, though in days gone by tuberculosis was also a frequent cause.

The presence of the enlarged gland is diagnosed by passing a probang down the oesophagus. If the enlarged gland or glands are constricting the oesophagus, then the head of the probang stops about midway through the chest cavity (1).

Another cause of the condition is an

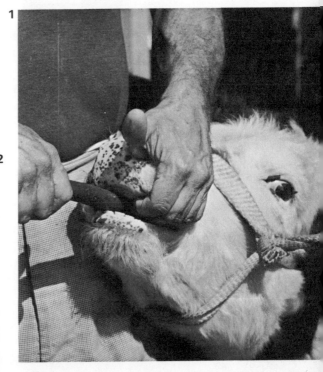

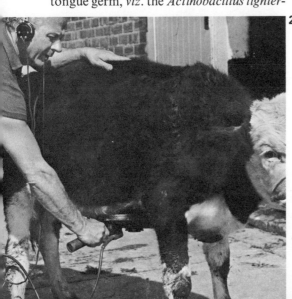

77

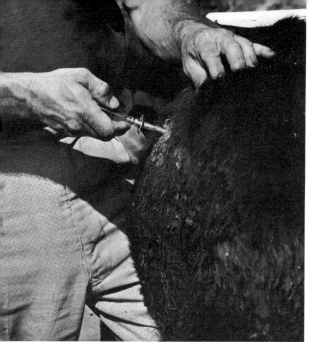

3 abscess formation or infection usually located at the junction of the second and third stomachs. Once again, the germ of wooden tongue is often involved and the resultant swelling and adhesions cause the bloat by interfering with the normal contractions of the second and first stomach.

Since the common cause of infection in this region of the digestive tract is wire, this possibility has to be eliminated by the use of the metal detector (2). The wire itself can also cause the same trouble by transfixing the far end of the second stomach.

4 Dilation of the fourth stomach or abomasum is another frequent cause. When the abomasum is dilated it feels like a bag full of watery fluid when the patient is pummelled in the right flank.

The final cause of recurrent bloat, and one which to my mind is much more common than a lot of people think, is hereditary weakness. Throughout the years I have come across several incurable cases, especially in Herefords and Hereford crosses, which showed absolutely no abnormality on *post-mortem* examination.

What To Do
Whether or not it is worth treating depends entirely on the animal's value. Mostly the answer is yes.

Treatment comprises approximately one week's hospitalisation. A cannula is inserted into the first stomach (3) and stitched into position to make sure that bloat doesn't occur during the night (4). And once the precise cause is determined the appropriate treatment is applied. If

5 wire is present it is removed. If infection of the glands or stomachs is suspected then a five- or seven-day course of antibiotic injections is given (5).

Unfortunately, recurrent bloat cannot be prevented; it is another condition which you have to deal with as and when it occurs.

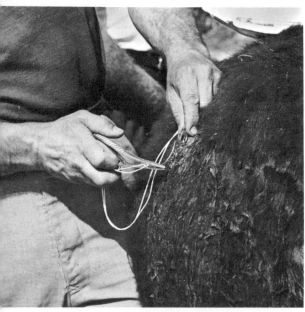

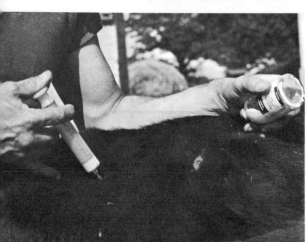

3
Displaced Abomasum

ONE of the recently discovered ailments of cattle is the condition known as 'displaced abomasum'. The abomasum is the fourth stomach of the bovine and normally it lies along the floor of the right-hand side of the abdomen. When displaced it usually passes underneath the rumen or first stomach and is found on the left flank or tucked up behind the left side of the rib-cage (1).

At one time this condition was never diagnosed and countless cattle must have been lost. Most veterinary surgeons, myself included, used to diagnose liver trouble and we never found the displacement at *post-mortem* examination simply because it usually righted itself when the stomachs were pulled out of the abdomen by the knackerman.

Breed Incidence
Although there is no certainty that it occurs more frequently in one breed than in any other, I have found it to be most common in the Channel Island breeds.

Cause
The specific cause is not known, but it is my opinion that the abomasum is displaced during the early stages of labour because displaced abomasum occurs nearly always in females and symptoms usually develop immediately after calving (2).

In normal pregnancy the calf is most often to be found on the right-hand side

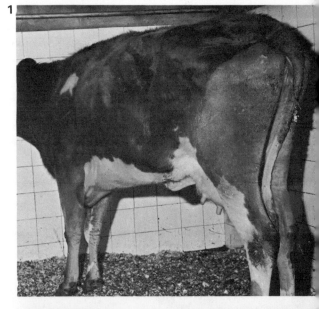

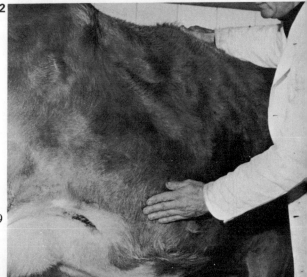

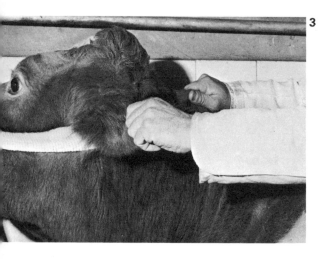

of the abdomen, and the front part of the womb bears pressure on the abomasum. I believe that the uterine contractions of labour, added to the weight and vigorous movement of the calf, are sufficient to push the abomasum underneath the rumen. This is most likely to happen when the cow is straining whilst lying on her right side. Of course, there must be other predisposing factors because the condition has

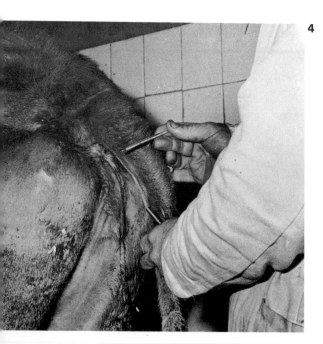

been reported in heifers and in bullocks. But whatever the cause, symptoms by and large appear after calving.

Recognising the Condition

Typically the affected cow is 'not herself' after calving. She may eat half heartedly for two or three days and then go off food completely for a similar period.

Her ears and/or horns may be alternately ice cold and warm or persistently cold (3).

She may be constipated or have intermittent attacks of diarrhoea, but her temperature is usually normal (4).

Because the cow has to exist largely on her own body fat, symptoms of acetonaemia may appear with the characteristic acetone smell in the breath (5) and milk.

Often, because of the cow's lowered resistance, an acute metritis (inflammation of the womb) may develop. This is characterised by an evil-smelling uterine discharge.

Two other less frequent symptoms I have observed are:

(1) Colic—repeated attacks associated with inappetence, and

(2) Shivering—again associated with periods of inappetence.

What To Do

In most instances a veterinary surgeon will be needed to make and confirm the diagnosis. Apart from observing the typical symptoms, he will confirm his suspicions by listening for the typical abomasum sounds in the left rib and flank region (6).

Personally I like to press sharply upwards underneath the left flank region, at the same time listening carefully for the typical tinkling abomasal sound (7). The sound has been described as identical to that produced by gurgling fluid some distance down a well or sewer. Certainly it is a characteristic noise—once heard never forgotten.

Having made the diagnosis, action must be decisive. If the animal is of little value and of a reasonable weight emergency slaughter might be considered. On the other hand, surgical treatment is virtually 100 per cent successful and should always be carefully considered, and promptly executed.

There are several surgical techniques, but the one I have found the most successful and the one now widely used is that performed under general anaesthesia (8).

The animal is first of all starved completely for 36 hours and water is withheld for the 12 hours immediately prior to the operation. This ensures that the abdomen is empty and enables the displacement to be rectified without excessive handling of the stomachs and peritoneum.

The cow is put down on the bed of the operating theatre with an intravenous injection of pentothal.

An intratracheal tube is passed into the wind-pipe and a 'cuff' on the tube is inflated to make it fit tightly. The end of the tube is now connected up to a closed circuit anaesthetic apparatus which induces and maintains a perfectly safe anaesthesia for as long as is required.

Another tube is passed into the cow's oesophagus or food passage in case the cow should regurgitate.

Surgery is performed with the cow propped on her back so that the weight of the first stomach and other abdominal contents will not interfere with the replacement.

The operation is extremely simple (9).

5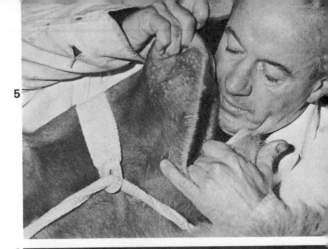

6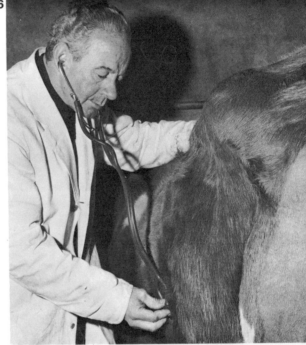

8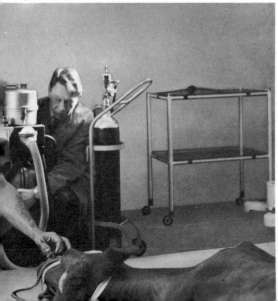

7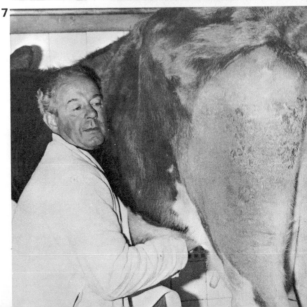

The abdominal cavity is opened up on the right-hand side of the mid-line (that is, where the abomasum should lie). The replacement is effected by introducing the hand and arm (coated with antibiotic cream) and lifting the stomach gently back into position.

The abomasum is anchored in its correct position by stitching its line of attachment to the peritoneum and first layer of abdominal muscle. The external wound is closed by two strong simple mattress sutures.

After Treatment

One of the most rewarding features of this operation is that almost invariably the patient starts to eat normally within 12 hours and a full ration of food should be given (10).

The external stitches can be removed after 10 days.

9

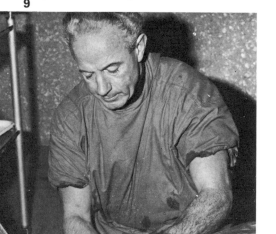

10

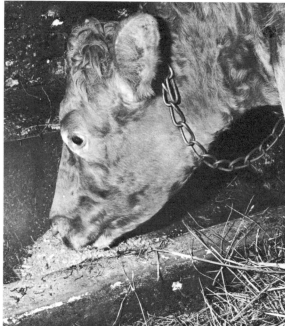

4
Dilated Abomasum

AN even more common condition than displaced abomasum is that of a dilated abomasum (1).

Cause

Indigestion caused by chronic inflammation or ulceration of the fourth stomach walls.

The irritation and ulceration frequently start in calfhood when they are caused by fibre getting through into the abomasum because the calf is not being fed often enough and in sufficient quantities to keep the fourth stomach full. The damage thus caused to the delicate lining of the abomasum can persist for a very long time.

Symptoms

The patient goes off her food. Her ears are cold and her motions may be stiff or, more often, diarrhoeic. The right flank often balloons out and when it is pummelled you can hear the dilated abomasum slopping about like a balloon full of fluid.

Treatment

Complete starvation for at least 24 hours —or as long as is necessary to reduce the abomasum to normal size. When this has been accomplished, diet the animal for at least a fortnight—small quantities of hay and good quality concentrates should be given four times a day.

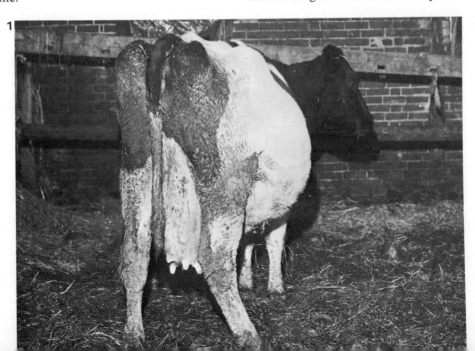
1

Surgery is contraindicated. I have opened and drained many a dilated abomasum but without any permanent success.

Torsion of the Abomasum

Just occasionally the dilated fourth stomach twists on its own axis. When this happens the cow becomes really ill with a weak thready pulse and distressed heart added to the symptoms of simple dilation. Such cases are hopeless and should be butchered immediately.

Obviously the diagnosing of a dilated or twisted abomasum is a job for a skilled and experienced veterinary surgeon. Subsequent treatment should always be under his supervision.

5
Wire or Foreign Bodies in Cattle
(Traumatic Reticulitis)

THIS condition affects cattle only. Despite the fact that the sheep has a digestive tract identical to that of the cow, wire cases are unheard of in the sheep. This is probably because the sheep's smaller mouth makes grazing and eating more selective.

Cause
Wire, nails, staples, flattened metal, sharp pieces of glass and even occasionally spicules of wood (1). These accumulate in the cow's second stomach which is called the reticulum. During the contractions of this second stomach the foreign bodies are caught up in the folds of the stomach lining and are pushed through the wall, piercing the peritoneum and passing either through the diaphragm towards the heart and lungs or downwards into the abdominal cavity towards the liver.

Where Foreign Bodies Come From
Chiefly from two sources—either the hay (2) or the corn. Occasionally nails or pieces of metal get into the concentrates before mixing and the hammer mill flattens them into bayonet-pointed killers (3).

Contrary to the general idea, it is only very rarely that a cow eats a foreign body whilst at grass. Veterinary surgeons know this by the fact that wire cases occur almost entirely during the winter when the animals are stall fed.

1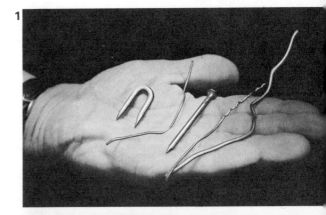

2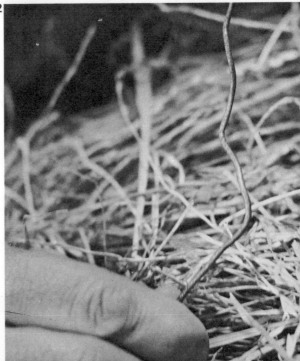

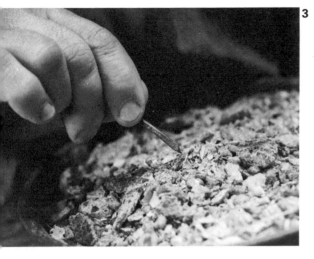

3 What Happens

Once it has been swallowed, the wire does not come up again with the cud because it gravitates into the second stomach or the reticulum and gets caught up in the folds of the lining (4). The wall of the reticulum is constantly contracting and the continual movements force the wire through the stomach wall, naturally causing the animal a great deal of pain and discomfort. The wire is forced either through the diaphragm towards the heart and lungs or downwards towards the liver.

As soon as the point pierces the outer covering of the stomach (5) a localised peritonitis is set up (*i.e.* an inflammation of the peritoneum, the fine glistening membrane which lines the entire belly cavity). It is this peritonitis which gives rise to the typical wire symptoms.

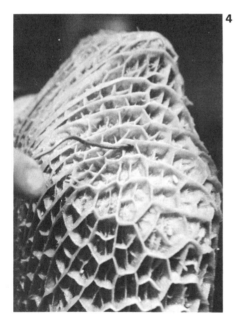

Symptoms

The most constant feature is a painful grunt which is accentuated when pressure is applied underneath the brisket where the second stomach lies against the diaphragm (6). When the pressure is applied, the patient will grunt, step back in the stall, and clearly evince pain in her eyes.

Another characteristic symptom is that the animal stops chewing the cud. She may continue to eat a little but she stops cudding. She is constipated and has a temperature of 103·4° to 103·6°.

The symptoms become more obscure in advanced or chronic cases. For example, when the wire touches the heart, it produces an inflammation of the membrane surrounding the heart, a membrane called the pericardium. This causes a collection of fluid or pus around the heart and sets up the condition known as *traumatic pericarditis*. Here the cow goes completely off her food, her ears and extremities become ice cold, and a dropsical swelling starts to develop underneath the brisket. The jugular vein in the neck becomes corded and prominent. A veterinary surgeon listening to the heart can usually diagnose the condition immediately.

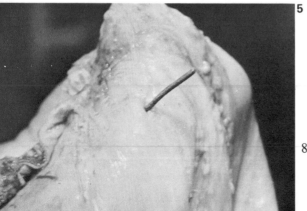

In other chronic cases abscesses may form in the liver and peritoneal cavity and produce obscure indefinable symptoms. From my experience, where one is presented with an obscure set of symptoms such as capricious appetite, unthriftiness and stiff walking in an adult cow or bull, then one should always suspect a foreign body.

The Metal Detector
The use of a metal detector is invaluable for only two purposes, first of all for confirming the typical symptoms and secondly and probably most important, to convince the farmer and persuade him into the expense of an operation (7).

It is wrong to use a metal detector indiscriminately because many foreign bodies, like nuts and bolts, have no sharp points and could stay in the stomach for years without causing the slightest trouble.

How To Treat The Condition
If the wire has touched the heart, the best treatment in the interests of economy and humanity is immediate slaughter. To date I have operated on 200 cases of traumatic pericarditis and only four have survived; in other words, the chances of success with surgical treatment after the wire has pricked the heart is no more than 2 per cent.

If, however, the symptoms are those of the typical traumatic peritonitis, then the only satisfactory treatment is the surgical removal of the wire (8). Undoubtedly many cases would settle down after five or six days without operation, but to let them do so is foolish since, apart from the ever-present danger that the animal may drop dead should the wire pierce the heart, the farmer, knowing the wire is there, has no further confidence in keeping her and in many cases sells her at a considerable capital loss.

There is no need to fear the operation; it is simple, straightforward and virtually 100 per cent successful, with complete

6

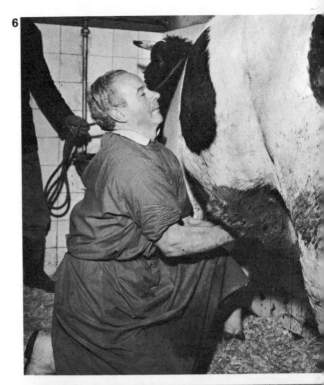

7

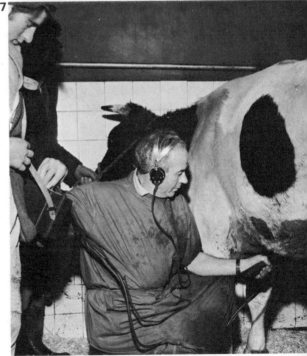

healing of the operation wound and return to normality in less than a fortnight.

How To Prevent Wire Cases

Complete prevention is impossible, but undoubtedly the use of string instead of wire in baling has done much to reduce the incidence.

Concentrates should be purchased from a reputable firm. If the farmer mixes his own ration, then everything possible should be done to prevent nails, etc., getting into the mixing. Recently a client of mine had the roof of his mixing shed repaired and subsequently I had to remove nails from 20 of his cows.

In Canada and America powerful cartridge-shaped magnets are fed to all cattle, the idea being that the wires and nails will cling to the magnet instead of piercing the stomach (9). Such an idea has much to commend it though proof of its efficacy has still to be produced.

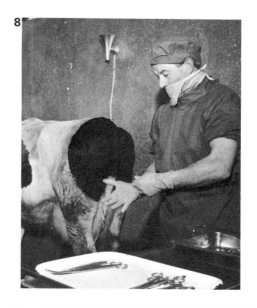

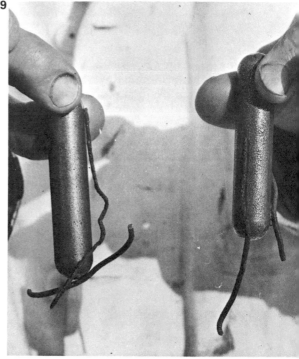

INTESTINAL DISEASE

Johne's Disease

JOHNE'S DISEASE is a world-wide problem. Although not very common in Ireland, it has been a very serious headache in Scotland, England and Wales for well over one hundred years.

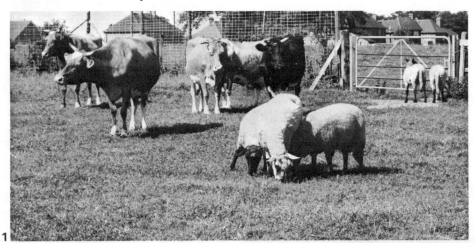

Animals Affected

Cattle, sheep and goats. It is important to remember that sheep are susceptible because it is possible for sheep to infect cattle and vice versa. It is my experience that few farmers associate Johne's disease with sheep (1).

Cause

It is caused by a germ which, in many respects, is similar to the germ which causes tuberculosis. It produces its effect by multiplying in the wall of the animal's intestine, thereby producing a chronic corrugated thickening of the bowel lining (2).

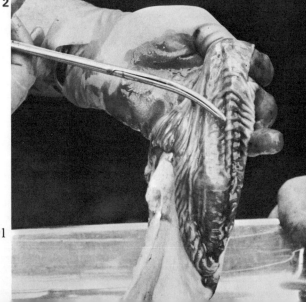

91

How Germ Is Carried

Active cases of the disease are the chief carriers of the Johne's germs but they are not the only carriers. Many healthy and apparently normal animals may carry the bug—as many as 17 per cent or even more.

The affected animals pass the germs out in their dung (3) and these germs thus contaminate the pasture, the feedingstuffs and the drinking water.

Outside the animal's body the Johne's germs can live for up to a year under suitable conditions.

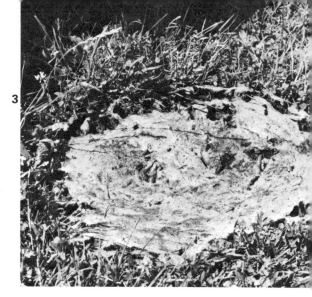

How Disease Develops

Some calves are born infected (4), having got the germ from the mother whilst in the womb (uterus). The majority, however, pick up the germs from contaminated teats or contaminated milk.

All available evidence seems to point to the fact that cattle are most susceptible to infection during the first two years of life. Any resistance-lowering factor during that vital growth period will predispose to the germ gaining a hold in the bowel wall, *e.g.,* calf scour, malnutrition or disease of any kind (5).

Once the germs gain a hold they proceed to multiply and very gradually to cause the chronic thickening. They require a very long time to produce the corrugated effect

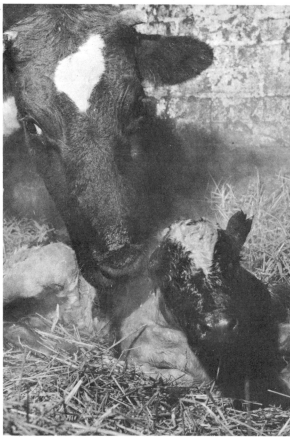

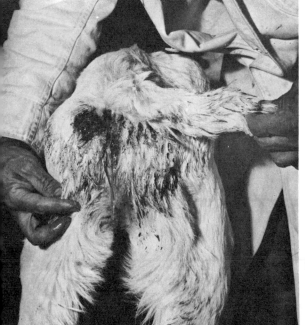

—one to several years—seldom less than two years.

This means that typical clinical signs of the disease mostly appear in animals from two to five years old. Once again any

92

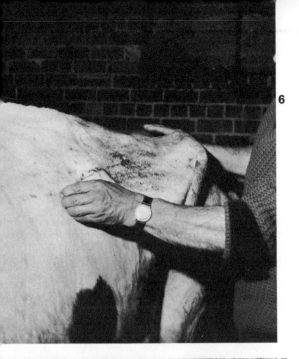

6

How To Recognise It

There is a characteristic unthriftiness and progressive loss in condition. This causes a tight, hidebound skin and a rough staring coat (6), despite the fact that the eye may still be bright and the appetite perfectly normal.

Occasionally a swelling appears under the jaw, but I always find that one of the earliest typical symptoms is the appearance of 'poverty lines' at the hind end (7).

The unthriftiness is associated with, or quickly followed by, intermittent or persistent dark-coloured and evil-smelling scour.

How To Detect Disease in Sheep

Symptoms in sheep are mostly disregarded and put down to parasitism. Diarrhoea is not a constant symptom though the dung may lose its characteristic pellet-formation for a time. Perhaps the only constant sign of Johne's disease in sheep is that of a progressive chronic wasting disease occurring in adult sheep when they are from three to five years old (8).

Confirming Presence of Disease

Microscopical examination of the dung is the most reliable and certain method of confirming the presence of the disease (9).

Blood samples can be taken, but the blood test is of value only when the

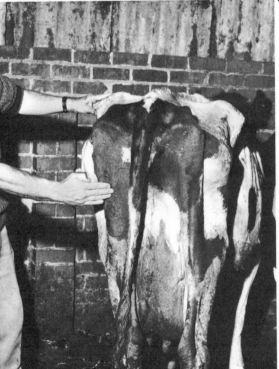

7

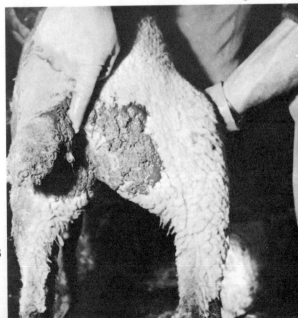

8

condition which markedly weakens the animals during that period appears to predispose to the disease flare-up. The most usual resistance-lowering factor in this group is the strain of calving.

clinical signs are well-developed and typical.

In sheep also, the only certain way of confirming the disease is by the laboratory examination of the dung.

Can It Be Treated?

The simple answer is no. Obviously, therefore, it is much better to concentrate on prevention.

How To Prevent It

A great deal can be done to control Johne's disease by simple commonsense husbandry.

I am convinced that if all young cattle during the first two years of their lives could be housed correctly and given an adequate diet, then the general incidence of Johne's disease could be reduced by at least 50 to 60 per cent. On many farms the young stock are undernourished during at least part of that vital growth period.

When the disease is really bad on the farm, the following husbandry routine will prove invaluable:

1. The calves should be taken from the dams immediately after birth and they should be reared in and kept in strict isolation (10). They should be suckled from sterilised stainless steel buckets. Of

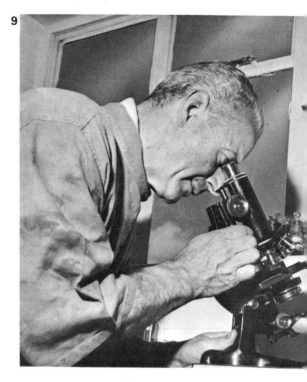

9

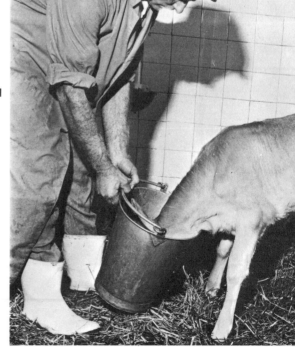

10

11

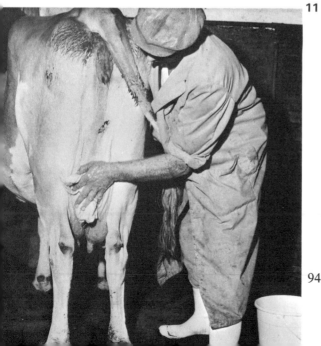

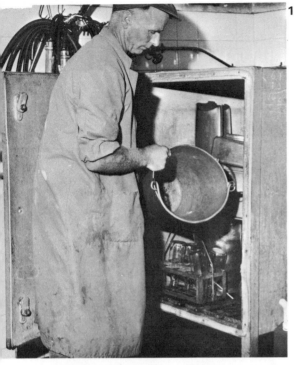

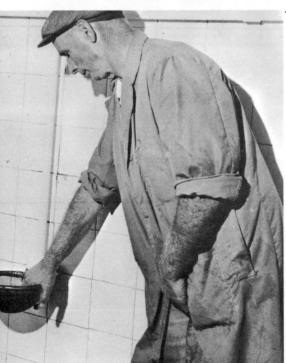

12 course, calves from cows showing clinical signs of the disease should never be reared because of the danger of their having been born with the infection.

2. Colostrum and milk fed to calves should come only from udders that have been thoroughly washed (11). In fact, if the herd infection is really severe, it is much better to feed a milk substitute.

3. Feeding utensils should be kept well clear of dung contamination and should be sterilised every day (12).

4. The calf's water and food supplies must also be protected from possible contamination by the dung of older animals (13).

5. Any cow showing signs of persistent or recurrent diarrhoea should be isolated at once and examined by a veterinary surgeon.

6. When Johne's disease is a problem, strip-grazing or paddock grazing must be avoided. Concentrated grazing means concentrated infection, and remember the bugs can live outside for up to a year (14).

7. If there are any drinking pits on the farm, they should be fenced off (15). 13 Drinking must be from troughs kept clear of dung contamination and supplied with fresh running water.

8. Drainage from cowsheds should never be allowed to flow on the pasture and manure should not be distributed on to grazing land (16).

14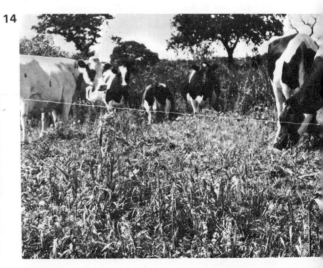

95

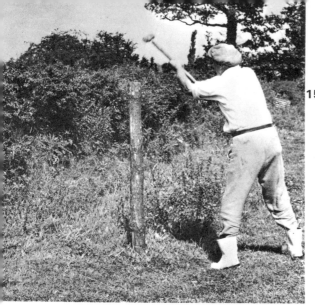

15

9. A first-class vaccine is now available for use in young calves. Because of the possibility that the vaccine may interfere with the tuberculin test, it is necessary, however, to get permission from the Ministry of Agriculture before using it (17).

On every farm where Johne's disease is a serious problem, all calves should be vaccinated under the age of one month. *This provides a solid protection and no further doses of vaccine need be given.* The intelligent use of this Johne's vaccine will save many lives and a great deal of money.

16

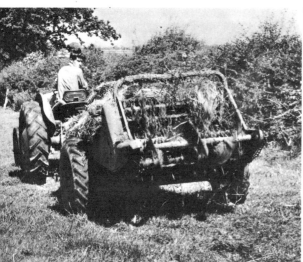

17

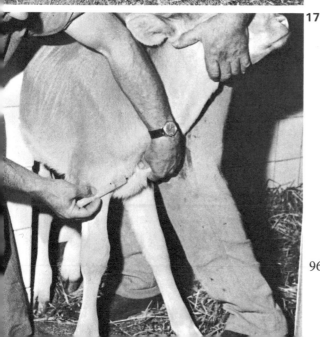

96

UDDER TROUBLES

1
Black Garget

IF there is one condition I hate to see it is black garget or as it is known technically, gangrenous mastitis. Apart from the fact that it is often fatal and difficult to treat, it invariably signals the beginning of the end for what is often the best milking cow in the herd (1). Rarely, if ever, do farmers keep three-quartered cows and the one thing certain about black garget is that it literally leaves a cow with three-quarters or even fewer simply because the affected quarter or quarters drop off altogether at variable times after the cow has apparently recovered her normal health.

Exactly the same thing happens in ewes, where most of the mastitis takes the form of black garget and there the condition is caused by the same germ found in cows—the dreaded *Staphylococcus*.

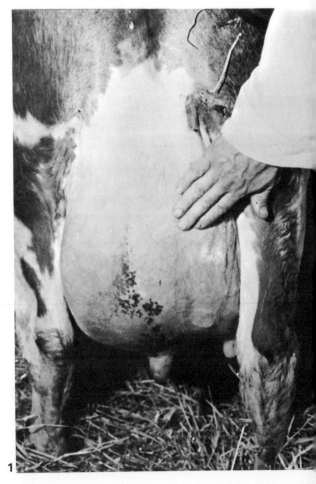

1

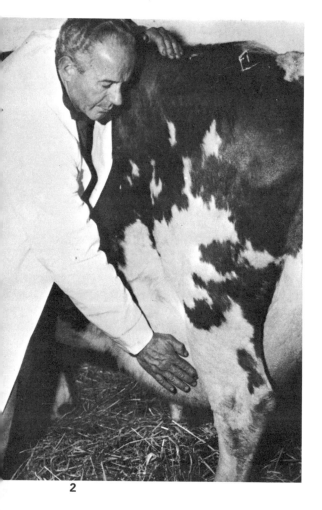

2

Where Germ Comes From

There are three sources:

(1) Inside the udder (2). In many cows the odd one or two staphylococci are normal residents of the udder, having got there from the cows' tonsils via the bloodstream. They lie dormant and cause no trouble unless or until the udder is damaged in some way.

(2) The surface of the skin of the teats and udder (3). Recent research has shown quite conclusively that the staphylococcus can live and grow on the skin surface. It doesn't cause any damage, of course, until it gains entrance into the tissue.

(3) The third source of the bug is the dried milk fat which is found in invisible cracks in the liners of the milking machine teat cluster (4). The germs will live there for a considerable time but again will cause no harm until the teats or udder are damaged in some way.

Cause of Disease Flare-up

Once again it is the old story of lowered resistance—scratches or cuts on the teats, damage to the teat linings caused by faulty milking technique, exposure to draught, etc.

Black garget is most commonly seen

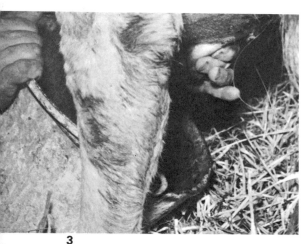

3

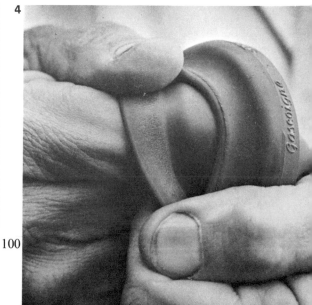

4

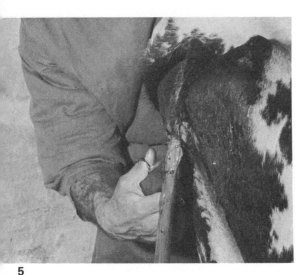

5

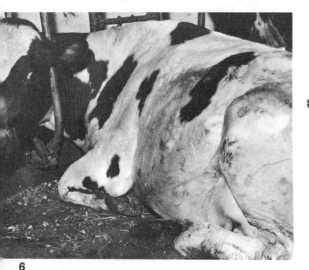

6

surface pits on pressure, *i.e.,* when the finger is pressed into it and removed a hole or pit remains (7).

The milk is bloody, often dark red, and it smells like the odour of sweet new bread (8).

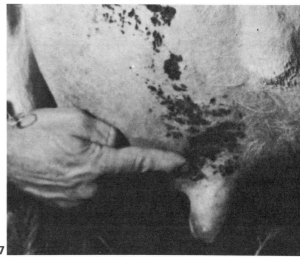

7

Occasionally there is profuse diarrhoea with the faeces black and watery.

I think it is important to know what to do with a case of black garget. *One thing is certain—there is no use having the cow*

8

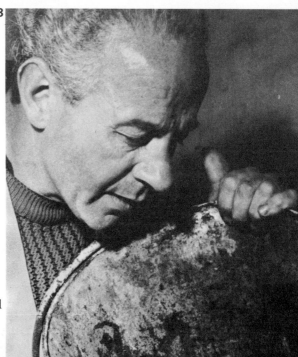

immediately after calving, especially when the afterbirth has been retained (5). In such cases the bug gains a hold simply because the calving and its sequelae sap the cow's reserves.

The first sign is usually unwillingness on the part of the cow to get up (6) and this, of course, is what makes many people suspect milk fever. The ears and extremities are ice cold and the temperature subnormal.

The affected quarter is swollen but may not be excessively so though usually its *slaughtered for salvage because all meat inspectors must by law condemn any carcase containing gangrenous issue.*

Treatment

The cases must be treated and it's surprising how well some of them respond. Massive doses of antibiotic injected into the muscle and udder (9) quickly control the invasion of the bloodstream. In fact, when death occurs it is more likely to be due to a toxaemia rather than a septicaemia, *i.e.,* to an excess accumulation of waste products or toxins excreted by the germs rather than an excess of the germs themselves.

Within 24 or 36 hours after commencing the treatment the cow will either die or suddenly get better in herself. In the cases that recover, what happens is that the gangrenous portion separates off from the healthy part of the body and the toxins are no longer absorbed into the bloodstream.

Despite the fact that the cows are no use for salvage I often have difficulty in persuading farmers to allow me to give treatment because, apart from the expense, they think they will be left with a non-productive animal. Also they don't fancy keeping the cow while the gangrenous quarter drops off. Certainly the sight and smell of the sloughing quarter is not very pleasant, but the cow quickly regains a milk yield in the normal quarters. And I have found it is quite safe to use the affected cow to suckle one, two or even three calves, depending on the number of quarters left and on the milking potential. In this way the cow will more than pay for her keep, and after rearing the calves, she can be fattened for the butcher or

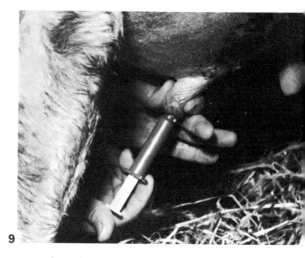

9

served again and kept solely for the job of calf rearing.

I would say, therefore, that it is always well worth having a case of black garget treated. The chances of successful treatment are probably around the 60 per cent mark, and within 48 hours the recovered cow can resume her useful economic life.

How To Prevent Black Garget

The rigidly correct milking technique recommended for the ordinary mastitis should always be strictly adhered to. One should be particularly careful to use a strong solution of chlorhexidine in the washing and drying water. The chlorhexidine will at least destroy the staphylococci on the udder surface.

Care should always be taken to dissolve the dried milk fat in the invisible cracks in the teat cup liners. This can be done by using two sets of liners, changing them each week and keeping the set not in use immersed in a 5 per cent solution of caustic soda.

2
Black Spot

THOUSANDS of first-class dairy cows are ruined by 'black spot' each year (1). It is, in fact, an insidious evil which many, if not all, dairy farmers have come to accept as inevitable throughout the years. When a case occurs they labour away with the antibiotic tube, with the teat syphon or with the bougies, and usually finish up with a three-quartered cow that soon finds its way into the barren ring.

But, despite its common occurrence, no one has as yet attempted to set down in print a simple explanation of the condition or some guiding principles in practical prevention.

Cause

It is caused by the identical germ which produces foul of the foot. The bug's name is *Fusiformis necrophorus,* but for our purpose the name is only of academic significance. To my mind it is much more important that we should understand exactly where the germ lives, where it comes from, and how it gets to work in the end of the teat.

Where Germ Comes From

The germ is a normal resident of the feet of most dairy cattle, living and persisting in the cracks between the wall and the sole (2). It comes out from its hiding place to contaminate the cow's bedding and the pasture. But it can live on pasture only for a maximum of 14 days, and it is unlikely to live on bedding for very much longer, though probably in cowsheds and in yards it does exist for around three weeks.

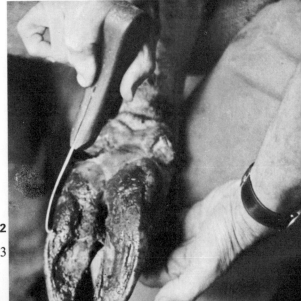

1

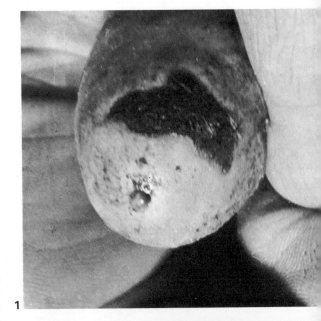

2

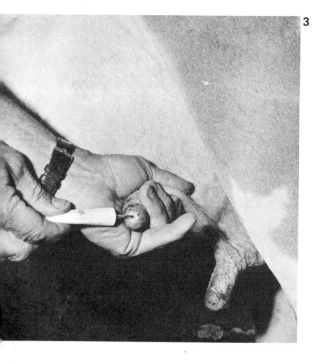

3 Obviously it stands a much better chance of surviving in damp, dirty conditions. And one of the frustrating facts is that as the germs die, fresh live bugs come from the feet to take their place.

How Germ Gets To Work

As in the case of foul in the foot, the germ has to gain entry through a wound before it can start to cause trouble and *the most common cause of traumatic wounds at teat ends is the rough insertion of the nozzles of antibiotic intramammary tubes* (3). Other wounds, of course, can be produced by crushing, but this generally occurs only in cowsheds and black spot is by no means a problem confined to dairy cows housed in byres.

Of course, wounds in the form of cracks can be produced on the end of the teats by repeated exposure of the udder to dirt and damp (4) and certainly such wounds do occur, particularly in yards bedded down with straw. *But in the main black spot is produced by the herdsman himself.*

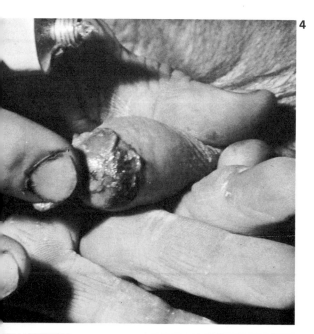

4 When the 'fusiformis' gets into the wound it multiplies and grows, and each germ excretes waste products or toxins which destroy the surrounding tissue producing necrosis or death. Black spot is, in fact, a lump of dead tissue which may extend some distance up the teat and which destroys the efficiency of the teat valve and eventually blocks the milk flow.

Treatment

It can be treated in the same way as 'foul of the foot', but such treatment is not nearly so spectacular in its result as in foul, simply because the blood supply in the teat end is not developed to anything like the extent as it is in the foot. Localised treatments (of which there are several) stand a much better chance of success and their application depends on the stage of lactation.

If the cow is in full milk and has been calved less than a month, then the best treatment is to have the end of the teat opened up by a veterinary surgeon (5) and thereafter to impregnate the affected area with antibiotic inserted, through the nozzle of an intramammary tube or syringe, twice daily for three days. Any additional external wounds on the teat should also be treated either with antibiotic cream or with dry sulpha powder.

If the cow has been calved more than a month, then I have found the plastic cannula the best treatment (6). The cannula is impregnated with a powerful antibiotic and should be left in position in the teat for a maximum of five days. Such cannulae are excellent and have saved many, many quarters, but if they are left in too long they tend to produce a 'cording' of the teat lining.

If the cow has been milking for a long time, then undoubtedly the best treatment of all is to fill the quarter with antibiotic once daily for three days (7) and leave the quarter to go dry. One of the more powerful antibiotics is best for this purpose. Subsequently, when the cow is newly milked, it may be necessary to re-open the teat but by that time the black spot will have disappeared, fibrous tissue will have taken its place and the teat operation will be completely successful.

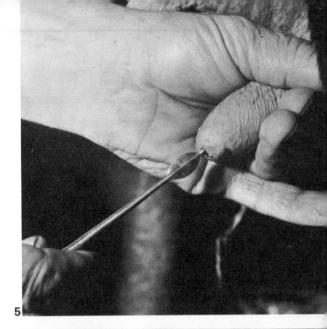

5

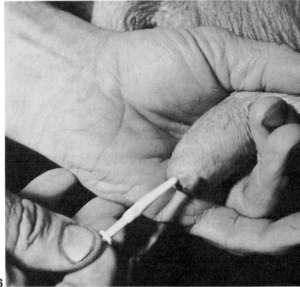

6

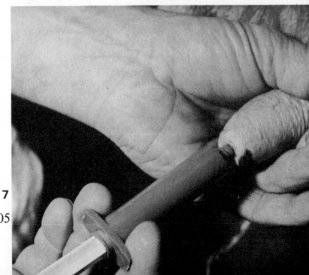

7

How To Prevent It

Prevention is simple—just take more time and more care when using intramammary antibiotics. Clean the end of the teat thoroughly (8) before inserting the nozzle —when this is not done live fusiformis bugs may and often do enter with the nozzle—and never force the end of the tube into the teat. Be patient—especially with heifers.

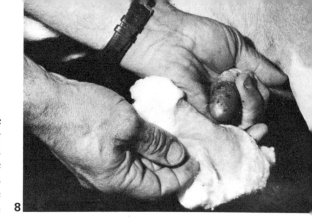

Wounds caused by dirt and damp are obviously easier to prevent in a cowshed than in a yard, and here the accent must be on simple cleanliness and good management. The beds should be swilled down thoroughly every day (9) and the rear portion of the bed (*i.e.,* where the udder is likely to lie) should be covered with sawdust (10).

Sawdust is also a great help in yards since it retains its dryness and cleanliness much longer than does straw.

In all dairy herds the cows' feet should be trimmed regularly—at least once every six months—particular care being taken to pare down the overgrown soles (11).

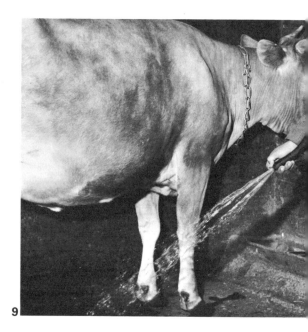

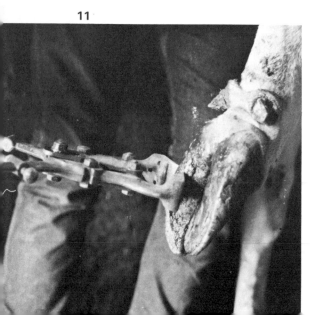

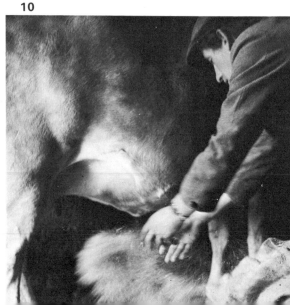

3
Mastitis

MASTITIS, which means simply inflammation of the udder, can be caused by a variety of different bacteria or germs. Clotted milk is nearly always the first sign (1).

Where Germs Come From
Practically all cowshed floors are reservoirs of infection. Mastitis germs are present on the surface of the skin of the udder and teats: in fact, one of the germs involved, the *Staphylococcus,* actually multiplies and grows there. Many more germs are already inside the udder waiting for their chance to multiply and produce mastitis. They get that chance when the udder tissue is damaged in any way.

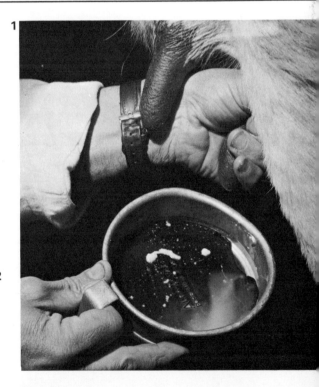

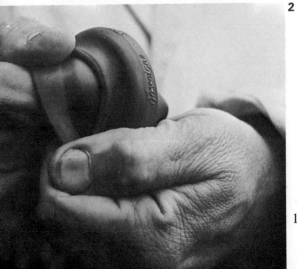

Another source of infection can be dirty teat cup liners. They accumulate skin fat and dried milk fat both of which can harbour germs in the invisible cracks in the rubber (2).

What Causes Damage To Udder Tissue?

The practical conditions that predispose to the modern mastitis problem in ascending order of importance are: *(a)* Feeding; *(b)* Housing; *(c)* Milking.

(a) Feeding

Steaming-up before calving produces a congestion and oedema of the udder (3) and renders the delicate udder tissue most susceptible to infection.

(b) Housing

Dirty, cold, damp floors, with little or no bedding, will lower the udder's resistance (4).

Inadequate space between the cows (5) can cause trouble with trodden teats.

Holes in the wall, broken windows, and ill-fitting doors direct draughts on to the udder and damage it in exactly the same way as does the dirty, damp floor.

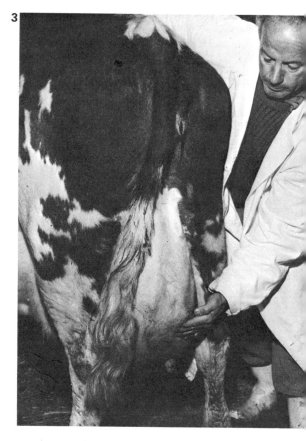

3

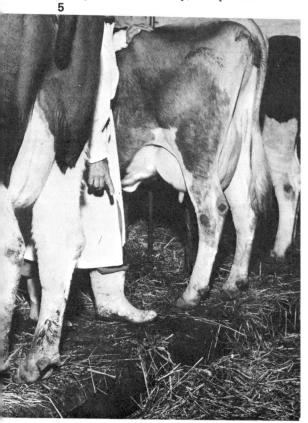

5

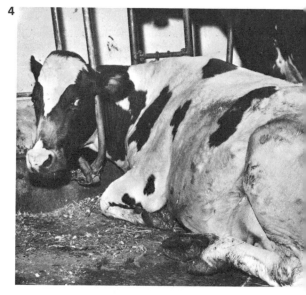

4

(c) Milking

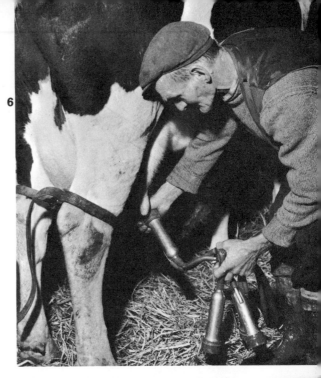

6

By far the most important predisposing causes of mastitis are to be found in the unskilled use of the milking machine (6).

The milk is let down one minute after the cow realises she is going to be milked and the let-down lasts only so long as there is milk in the udder and then only for a maximum of around seven minutes. In unskilled milking, if the units are put on too quickly (that is, within the minute), the clusters draw the delicate lining of the milk cisterns into the teats and bruise and damage it, at the same time injuring the lining of the teats (7).

The same thing happens when the units are left on too long. The germs move in on the damaged lining, multiply, grow and produce a severe mastitis.

Inconstant vacuum pressure can cause trouble (8). Low vacuum pressure means slow milking, and high vacuum pressure can cause teat erosion. Variations in

7

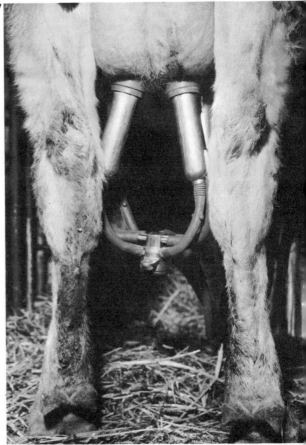

8

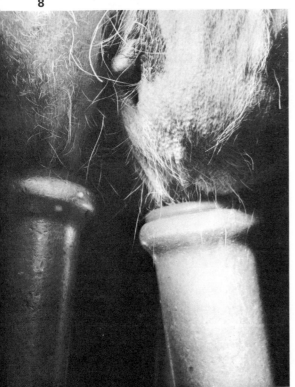

pulsation and worn-out teat liners can also cause teat erosion (9), both inside and out.

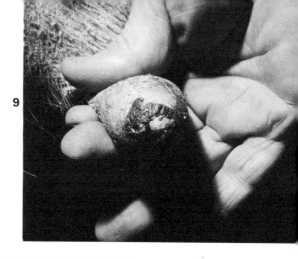

How To Eliminate and Control Mastitis

Obviously each outbreak should be treated as an individual herd problem and that means getting a veterinary surgeon to conduct a comprehensive on-the-spot investigation, which should enable him to pinpoint the faults. However, the complete general routine is as follows:

The liners. Use one-piece moulded, high-tension, pure rubber liners and use two sets of liners for each cluster. Change them each week and keep the set not in use immersed in a 5 per cent solution of caustic soda (10). This will de-fat the liners and destroy the germs.

Examine the liners carefully each time they are used (11) and ruthlessly discard and replace when necessary.

The vacuum pressure. Have the vacuum pressure checked and adjusted by a skilled engineer at least once every three months.

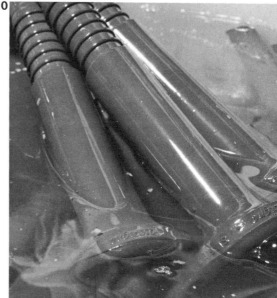

There should be absolutely no variation of pressure while the units are being changed from cow to cow, even if ten units are on the go. The usual pressure recommended in the bucket plant is 13 to 14 p.s.i. (12).

Pulsation. Check the pulsation regularly. Provided they are constant, pulsation

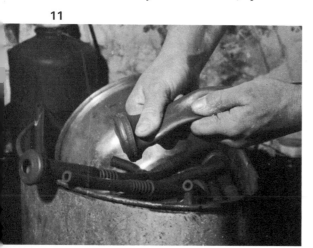

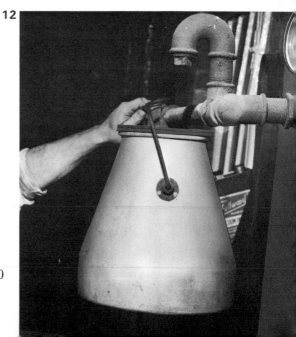

speeds can be stepped up, with advantage, to between 48 and 60. Perhaps for constancy the master pulsator with subsidiary slave pulsators (13) is the nearest to the ideal although it is not by any means essential.

Milking technique. Organise the labour so that one man should work only two and the same two units all the time; using the strip cup, washing, drying and milking, but not feeding or carrying milk. A competant man can milk a herd quicker with two units than with four (14).

Use two buckets and two differently coloured cloths for washing and drying. This keeps everything clean longer because the drying cloth is always returned to comparatively clean water (15).

Use plenty of really hot water (16) and replace after every ten cows. *It is vital to add the recommended amount of a reliable udder antiseptic. In my opinion, an udder wash containing chlorhexidine is the most satisfactory because this drug will destroy the staphylococci on the teat and udder surface.*

Always use the strip cup even if the herd is comparatively clear. An early diagnosis

13

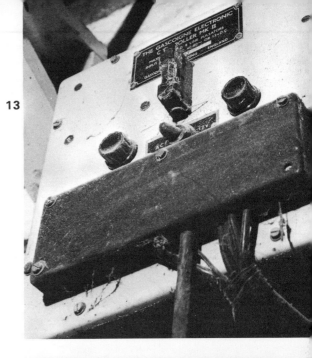

14

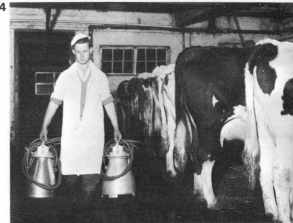

16

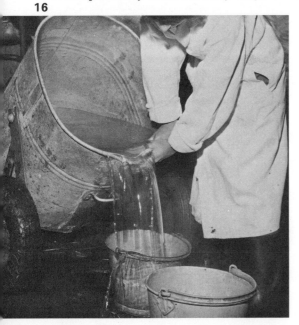

15

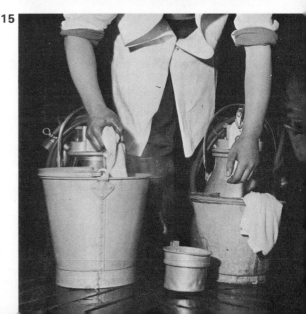

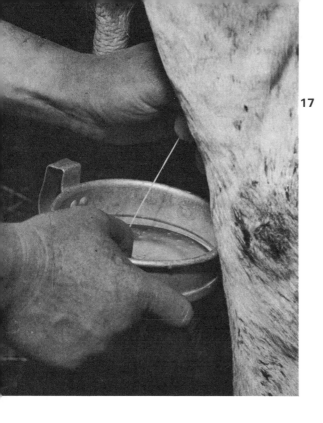

17

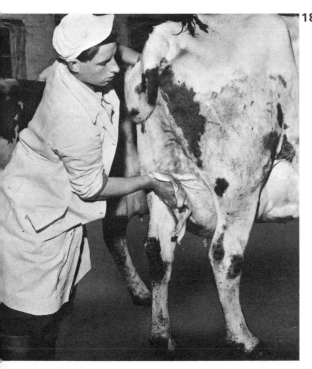

of trouble can make all the difference to control (17).

Now the washing. Thorough washing and drying are essential, but the technique should be developed so that as near as possible only one minute elapses between the start of the washing and the putting on of the clusters because at one minute the milk let-down is at its greatest and best (18).

A correct routine can soon be acquired, but it is a good idea to time the process during a few successive milkings. Check on a borrowed stop-watch or install a clock in the shed.

Since the average cow in the herd will give only 20 or 30 lb. of milk, two or three minutes should be all the time necessary for milking. For this reason the cowman should always be on hand from two minutes onwards ready to finish off the cow (19). Only when working two units is this possible.

Finish the cow by pressing gently on the base of the cluster for a maximum of 20

18

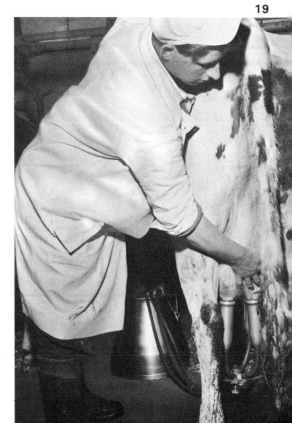

19

seconds. This prevents any tendency for the cups to creep up the teats and at the same time effectively strips the quarters (20). Don't worry about the last drop, leaving a small quantity of milk in the udder will never cause mastitis.

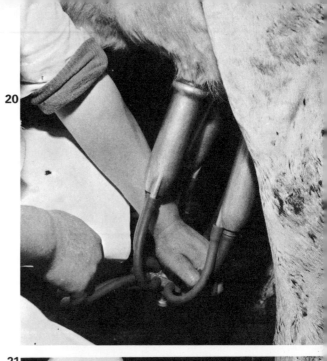

After removing the cluster, dip each teat in one of the non-irritant teat dips. This is a most important factor in control.

If the cluster should fall to the floor during milking, always dip it in a solution of chlorhexidine before moving to the next cow (21).

Correct milking technique can be summed up by saying that rapid milking is efficient and essential to udder health. Over-milking is injurious and ever liable to throw up a case of mastitis.

Treatment of active cases is, of course, by the insertion into the udder of various antibiotics, but it is most unwise to rely on these. Wherever there occurs persistent mastitis the veterinary surgeon should be consulted at once. Quite apart from investigating and recommending a control routine, he can type the germ involved and prescribe a specific cure when necessary.

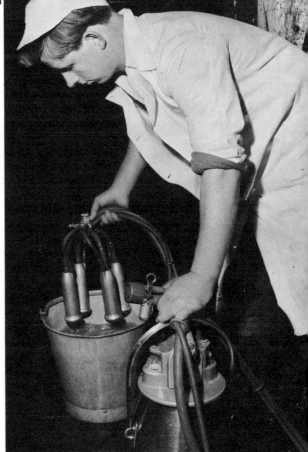

With parlour milking now in vogue, the cowman has to handle more and more cattle in less and less time. Inevitably the incidence of mastitis is on the increase. In parlours, therefore, precautions should be unlimited. I recommend a single udder cloth for each cow and rubber gloves to be worn by the herdsman; plus a routine insertion of long-acting antibiotics into the teats of every cow as it is dried off.

Dry Cow Therapy
The drug 'Orbenin' is probably the best of the long-acting antibiotics (22).

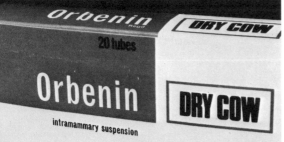

4
Summer Mastitis

SUMMER MASTITIS (1) is known by many different names —'August Bag', 'Garget', 'Felon' and so on. It affects chiefly dry cows and occurs usually during July, August and September.

Cause

The germ chiefly associated with the disease is called the *Corynebacterium pyogenes,* a germ which is a normal resident of the tonsils of every cow.

Every now and then, one or maybe two of the *C. pyogenes* germs get into the blood stream and are carried to the udder. There they stay, doing no harm at all as they cannot grow or multiply until they

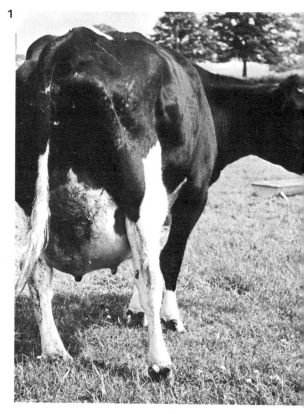

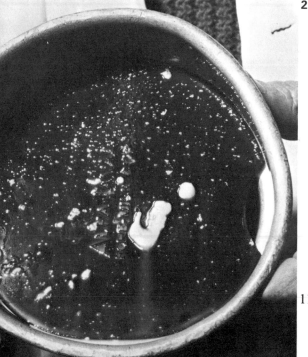

have a suitable base to grow on such as damaged tissue. The damage must be reasonably extensive since the multiplication of the *C. pyogenes* does not start easily (2).

The dry cows, with the odd one, two, or several inactive summer-mastitis germs in their udders, are turned out to pasture. In the fields, especially those surrounded by trees or high hedges, and particularly in the hot moist thundery weather of late July and August, the fly population is at its height. As a result very often the cows' teats become covered with black masses of flies.

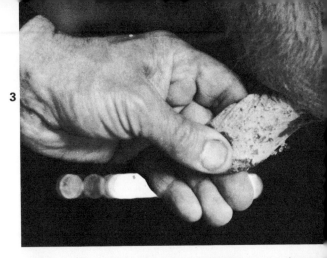

A close look at the surface of such teats reveals a mass of tiny red fly bites (3). This superficial damage allows the common mastitis germs, usually the *streptococcus agalactiae,* to multiply and grow in the udder producing a simple streptococcal mastitis.

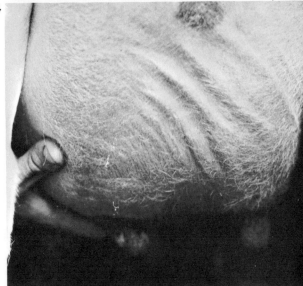

The streptococci may gain entrance through the wounds caused by the flies, but more often they are ordinary residents of the udder, having reached there in much the same way as the summer mastitis germ —from the tonsils via the blood.

The *C. pyogenes* germ now seizes its chance. The extensive tissue damage caused by the streptococcal mastitis presents an ideal medium for its propagation. By multiple division one million germs form from a single germ inside 24 hours. All these million-odd germs excrete waste products called toxins. The toxins destroy the damaged tissue, causing an intense and painful hardening of the udder (4).

Some of the toxins may be absorbed into the bloodstream causing the cow to be very ill. They make her go off her food, blow hard and sometimes they put her right off her legs. Then, as most of us say, 'the poison is in the cow's system'.

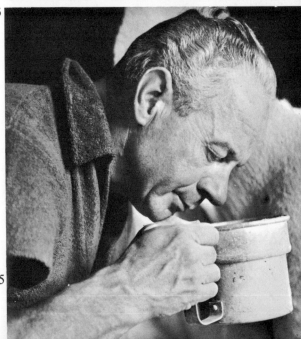

At this precise stage there is no smell from the teat contents. Still another germ is concerned in the production of the typical evil smell associated with summer mastitis. This germ is a gas-producing streptococcus called an *anaerobic streptococcus.* It attacks the dead tissues produced by the *C. pyogenes* toxin and causes putrefaction. The putrefaction gives rise to the typical smell (5). Then and only then, do you have a typical summer mastitis.

115

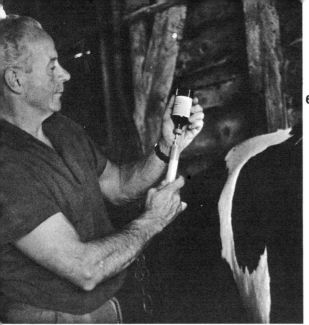

6 How To Recognise It

You can tell that it is summer mastitis by the season of the year and the fact that the cow is usually dry. But, most of all it is recognised by the typical putrid smell of the teat contents. The cow may or may not have a high temperature.

What To Do

Treatment is very much a job for the veterinary surgeon. He will prescribe a course of toxoid injections which will prevent the poison spreading and save the cow (6–7). Rarely, if ever, however, is it possible to save an affected quarter once the typical smell has developed. Nevertheless, if the cow is close to calving, it may be worthwhile trying one of the more powerful intramammary antibiotics.

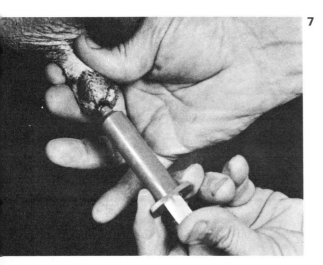

7 How To Prevent It

1. Have as few cows as possible dry during the vital period, *i.e.,* July, August and September.
2. Keep all dry cows with the milkers in 'open' fields and bring them in with the milkers twice daily. I say 'open' fields because fields surrounded by trees or high hedges have a very big fly population.
3. Insert into each teat of each dry cow towards the end of June and once a fortnight thereafter to the end of August, one long-acting antibiotic tube (8). This will maintain a concentration of antibiotic in the udder and will prevent the growth of the primary 'trigger' streptococcus. *Without this trigger streptococcus the C. pyogenes germ will not grow.*

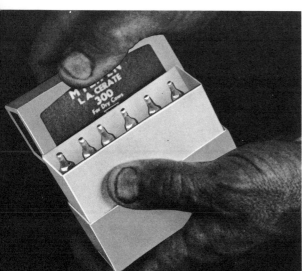

   Long-lasting antibiotics, that persist in the udder for a month, are now available. They are expensive but well worth it, especially if the resident mastitis germ is a powerful one ('Orbenin' – dry cow therapy).
4. Inspect the udders of the dry cows at

least once a day and coat the entire teats with collodion. Concentrate on the teats since the udder skin is thicker and not so vulnerable. The collodion forms a protective skin (9).

Alternative dressings that may be used are concentrated anti-fly solution (10) and Stockholm tar (11). The anti-fly solution does not prevent the flies biting but it does prevent them staying any length of time on the treated surface. The Stockholm tar, especially in the hot weather, may irritate or burn the teat skin.

5. Summer mastitis can and does occur in

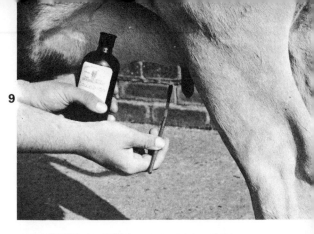

9

heifers, both maiden and in-calf heifers. The only thing that can be done to prevent the disease here is to run the maiden and in-calf heifers on short pasture during the vital months. Excess grass causes premature flushing of the udder and this undoubtedly predisposes to infection.

6. Fortnightly injections against the germ may be used but these are expensive and of doubtful value.

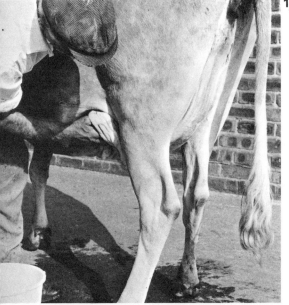

10

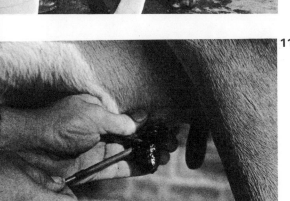

11

FOOT TROUBLES

1
Abscess in the Foot

A PICKED-UP nail (1) or a punctured wound of any description, which happens if any foreign body penetrates the hard sole, nearly always introduces infection to the sensitive tissues underneath. When it does so, abscess formation is inevitable.

How To Recognise Condition
Acute lameness occurs, without any external signs of swelling or pain. Severe pain is manifested when the affected claw is hit sharply with a hammer or with the handle of a knife, *etc.* (2).

What To Do
As in the case of the stone in the foot, abscesses can only be located by very careful searching. Because of this, it is always best when an abscess is suspected to call the veterinary surgeon. He will search for the tell-tale black mark which usually indicates the point of entry of the foreign body. He will cut right in boldly and release the pus. Afterwards he will enlarge the hole sufficiently to allow adequate drainage.

If you want to do this job yourself, then as soon as the abscess is tapped (3) an

1

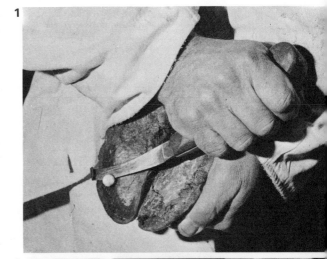

2

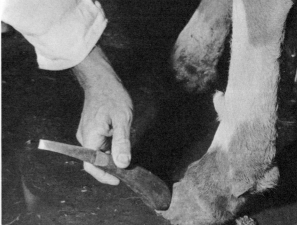

extremely sharp knife has to be used to enlarge the abscess cavity by cutting the hard sole from within outwards (4). If you attempt to continue cutting inwards, bleeding will soon obscure the field and prevent a decent job being made.

After-treatment

When a sizeable hole has been made to drain an abscess cavity, it is essential that the entrance should be kept open and clean for at least a week. This not only allows correct drainage, but also gives the horn a chance to grow over the hole. The foot should be bathed, therefore, in hot water and antiseptic once daily.

Between each bathing, the foot should be covered with a sack to prevent grit from the floor blocking the abscess cavity and gaining entry between the hard and soft sole (5).

Abscesses can be prevented to some extent by cleaning up the pastures as recommended in the prevention of 'foul'.

3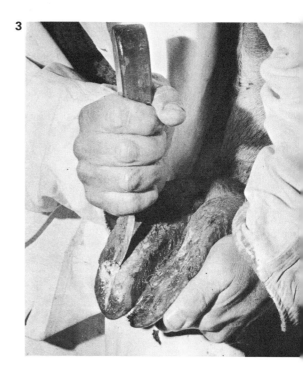

5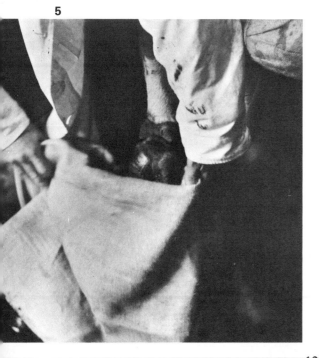

4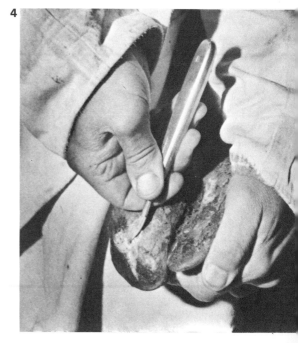

2
Digit Amputation

OCCASIONALLY, a neglected foul in the foot is complicated by a secondary bacterial invasion of a joint or bone (1).

The secondary abscess, unable to drain properly from underneath, penetrates inwards until it reaches and involves either the bone or the joint (2).

How To Recognise Condition
An acute painful swelling particularly just above the coronet (3). Pressure in this region causes violent reflex from the cow. The affected animal is obviously in severe pain. In many cases she shivers or refuses to stand and invariably there is a rapid loss in condition.

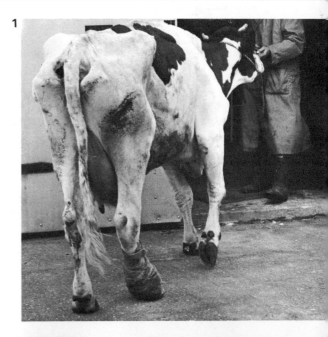

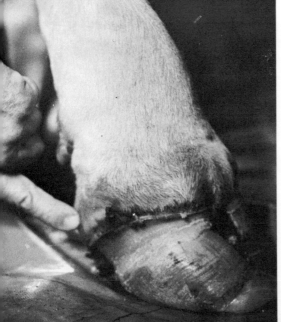

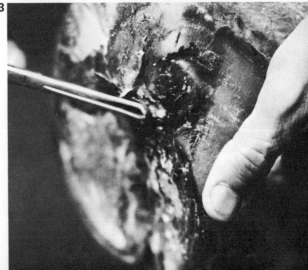

What To Do

This really is a job for the veterinary surgeon. An X-ray may be necessary to confirm the bony damage. Once it is established that the joint or bone are affected, then an operation is absolutely essential (4–5).

The operation is highly successful and economical. One digit is removed completely thus taking away all the infected tissues. Afterwards the cavity is packed with antibiotics and sulpha drugs, covered with sterile gauze, bandaged up, and left for as long as the dressing will stay on (6)—usually about five weeks.

Long before the end of that time the cow will be walking quite sound and a stump of horn will be growing over and protecting the raw surface. The horn grows from the coronary band (around the top of the foot) which is left on during the dissection.

The operation is performed under a general anaesthetic.

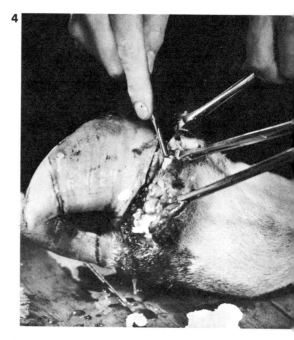

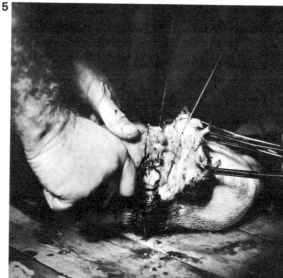

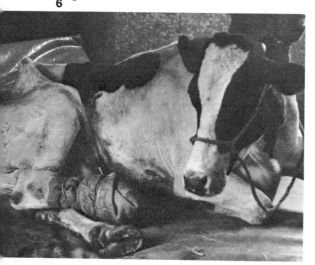

3
Foul in the Foot

FOUL IN THE FOOT is caused by a germ called the *Fusiformis necrophorus*.

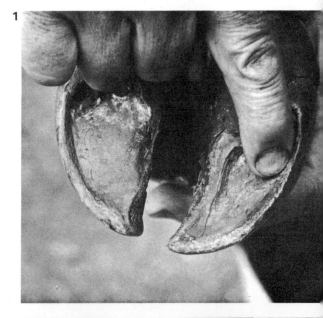

Where Germ Comes From
The germ can and does live for years in cracks and crevices in the cow's feet (1). On the pastures or in the dung, the fusiformis can live only for a maximum of three weeks.

What Causes Flare-up?
The important thing to remember is that 'foul' germs cannot grow or cause any trouble at all until they find a suitable place to grow in. The ideal place is a wound such as an abrasion, cut, or crack in the skin between the claws or around the bulbs of the heels.

The wounds may be caused by a piece of stone or gravel getting in between the claws or by pieces of wire, wood, metal or glass (2).

But perhaps the most constant predisposing factor is the repeated soaking of the feet in mud, water, dung, or urine. Muddy areas around drinking troughs and gateways are constant sources of danger, as are wet and stony collecting yards or even inadequately bedded straw yards.

Once the fusiformis gains entry into a wound, it starts to multiply rapidly causing, first of all, a painful swelling and then later death of the part affected. The

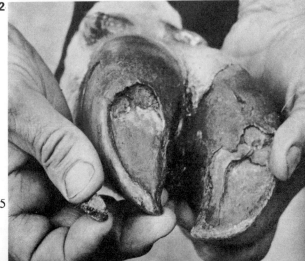

125

dead tissues (3) give rise to the character-istic 'foul' smell.

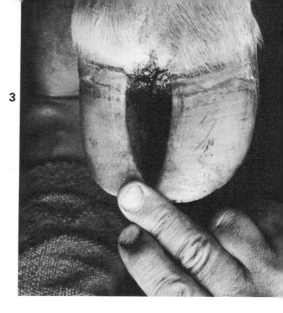

3

If the condition is not treated promptly, other germs move into the area and cause secondary septic complications any one of which may lead to an infected joint.

How To Treat A Case

It is most important that there is an accurate diagnosis as there are so many things that can produce lameness. For this reason it always pays to let your veterinary surgeon make that diagnosis. Treatment may comprise the subcutaneous injection of a fairly large quantity of a specific sulpha drug (4), and unless this injection is done correctly, abscesses may develop, which will prove more troublesome than the original 'foul' infection. Antibiotic injections are also spectacularly success-ful provided the diagnosis is correct.

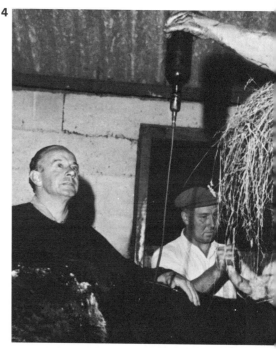

4

How To Prevent 'Foul'

Since it is not possible to kill all the germs living in the cow's feet, the obvious next best thing to do is to try to keep the germs from growing by eliminating the factors which cause the wounds and cracks. This is just common sense.

First of all, the grazing land should be combed and cleared of all stones, sticks, pieces of metal, wire, glass, *etc*. This is nothing like as difficult as it sounds. Three men walking systematically can clear most of the pasture land within a day or two, especially at the back-end of the year when the fields are comparatively bare.

The next job is to set about concreting the yards and gateways and the muddy areas around the drinking troughs (5). This is not an expensive job if you use your own labour and buy materials direct.

Next get your veterinary surgeon to supply you with a really first-class set of foot clippers. With these, in the early spring and again at the back-end, trim the feet of all the cows (6).

It's not enough to trim the toes off. A sharp knife must be used to get the under

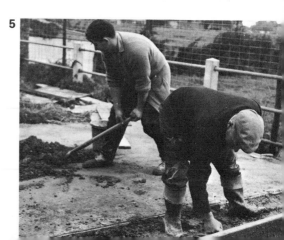

5

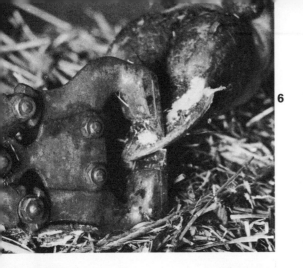

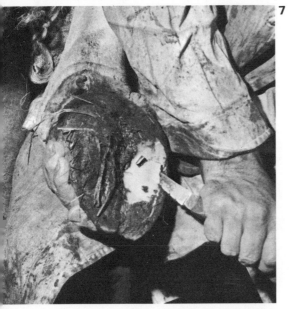

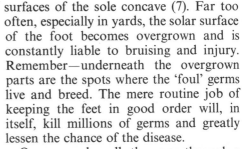

6

7

8

surfaces of the sole concave (7). Far too often, especially in yards, the solar surface of the foot becomes overgrown and is constantly liable to bruising and injury. Remember—underneath the overgrown parts are the spots where the 'foul' germs live and breed. The mere routine job of keeping the feet in good order will, in itself, kill millions of germs and greatly lessen the chance of the disease.

Once a week walk the cows through a foot bath containing a 3 per cent solution of copper sulphate or a 10 per cent solution of formalin (8). Afterwards, leave the herd in the yard for an hour or so for the feet to dry out. This will destroy some of the germs, but more important it will harden and toughen the skin in the vital areas. A foot-bath can be improvised by blocking a drain and making an artificial pool in the corner of the yard.

Every day, walk the cattle over a thin bed or a heap of ordinary lime. The lime keeps the skin over the heel areas hard and dry. The lime bed should extend right across a part of the yard over which each cow is certain to walk at least once a day. This is an extremely simple tip but I can assure you it is most effective.

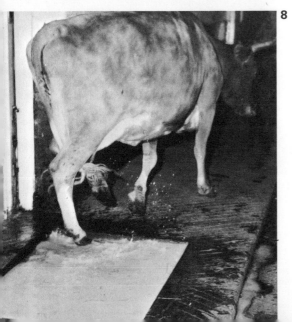

4
Stone in the Foot

ON farms where cows have a fair amount of road-work a piece of chipping is often picked up by the foot. This chipping works its way gradually through the sole into the underlying 'quick' or sensitive tissues.

As soon as the chipping starts to bear on the sensitive 'quick', it causes acute lameness.

How To Diagnose The Condition
The simplest and surest way of detecting which claw is affected is to strike the soles sharply either with a hammer (1) or with the handle of the knife. If there is something there, the cow will kick violently or show some other violent pain reaction.

Next a careful search of the foot, using a strong sharp foot knife. All suspicious black areas must be followed right down (2).

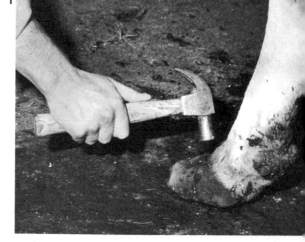

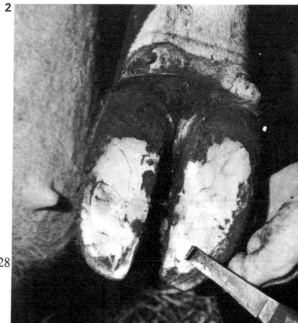

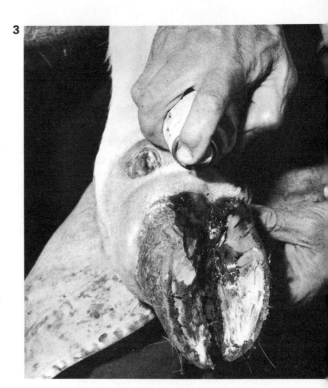

What To Do
Cut all the horn away from around the stone and lever it out with the point of the knife. Fill the cavity left with antibiotic or antiseptic (3) and keep the foot covered over with a sack for at least four or five days. If in any trouble, send for your veterinary surgeon.

GENERAL DISORDERS

1
Choke

ONE of the emergencies likely to occur during the winter feeding of stock is choke (1). A potato or piece of mangold gets firmly lodged in the top of the cow's oesophagus.

Symptoms

The symptoms are unmistakable: the animal slobbers from the mouth and coughs incessantly. If tied up, she will run back on her chain repeatedly and pass small quantities of urine and dung. She may blow up markedly and rapidly in the left flank.

Treatment

The first thing to do is to 'phone for a veterinary surgeon, but whilst waiting for

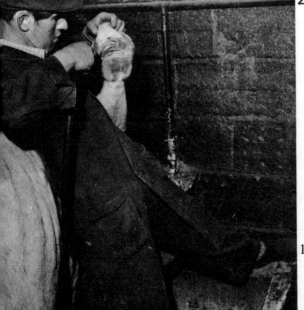

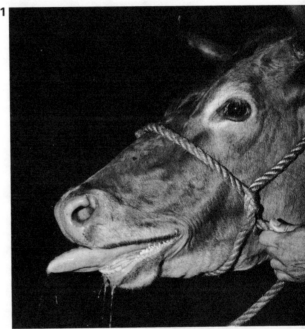

him there is just one intelligent first-aid remedy that can be tried and that is the manual removal of the foreign body.

On no account should attempts be made to push the potato or mangold down with a milking pipe (2) or a broom handle. It seems remarkable that anyone should be foolish enough to try pushing a broom handle down a cow's throat, but I have seen this happen several times with disastrous results. The end of the pole is forced through the back of the pharynx and this leads to death of the animal.

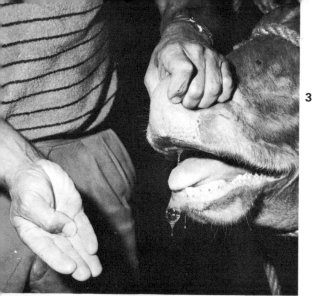

3 If the bloat condition becomes alarming, an emergency puncture may be necessary. (See chapter on BLOAT.)

Manual Removal

First of all, with an assistant holding the animal's horns or ears, grab hold of the nose with the left hand. It is essential that the person attempting the removal should hold the head himself so that he can anticipate the head movements and keep his hand and arm from being ground between the molar teeth. Now cup the right hand into the smallest size possible (3).

4

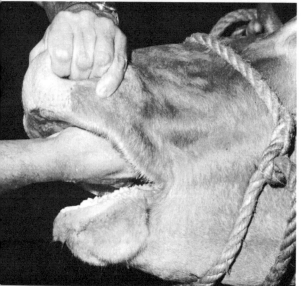

Introduce the right hand into the mouth and immediately press the palm upwards and firmly against the cow's hard palate and between the upper molar teeth. Move the hand carefully from side to side to make sure the molars are bilateral (4).

Keeping the palm of the hand tightly against the hard palate slowly push the hand towards the back of the throat. As the animal's head twists and turns, as it will do, the position of the right arm and hand can be synchronised by the control exerted on the nose by the left hand (5).

At the back of the throat pass the hand over the epiglottis into the oesophagus which is the top passage leading from the pharynx. Turn the hand round and grasp the offending piece of potato or mangold with the fingers. Then once again turn the palm, this time enclosing the foreign body hard against the roof of the mouth and gradually withdraw it (6).

5

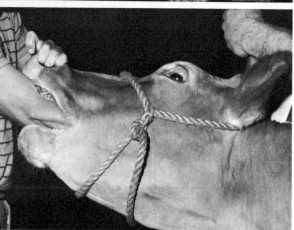

6

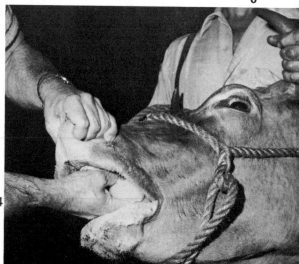

The animal's relief will be immediate and apparent, but the way to test whether the obstruction has been removed without damage is to offer some food—if the animal eats, then it is completely better (7).

The veterinary surgeon may have to push the obstruction down with a special probang (8), but this is a highly skilled and dangerous job and should never be attempted by the farmer.

Prevention

If feeding whole potatoes, feed them either small or large (9). *The medium-sized potato is the danger.* The small ones can be swallowed safely and the large ones have to be chewed. Mangolds should always be fed chopped.

Another preventative hint well worth trying is to feed the potatoes from the ground instead of from troughs. This prevents gulping and will certainly reduce the incidence of choke.

7

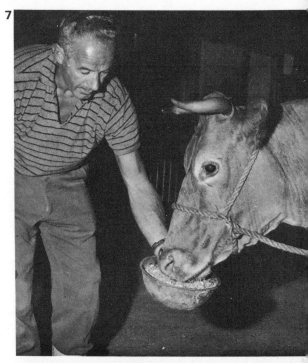

9

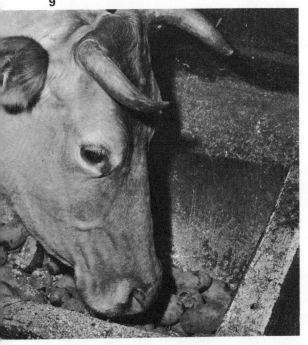

8

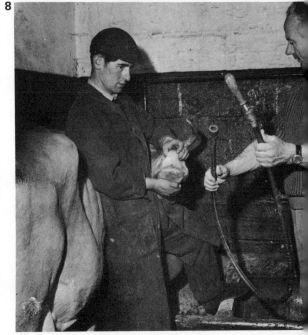

2
Big Legs

IN cattle practice I find that there are two common 'big leg' conditions.

First, the allergic type (1). This usually affects one or both forelegs, though I have seen all the legs involved.

Cause
An allergy, usually dietetical and often associated with a young fresh clover root.

Symptoms
These appear suddenly. The affected leg or legs are swollen, oedematous, and painful to the touch. Clear serum often exudes from the surface (2).

The animal may or may not run a temperature or go off food.

Treatment
Injections of cortisone or antihistamine (3) and a change of diet for a week produce a spectacular recovery.

The second type is seen chiefly in the hind legs and normally only one is affected (4).

Cause
The precise cause of the trouble is a germ called the *Corynebacterium pyogenes*—

1

2

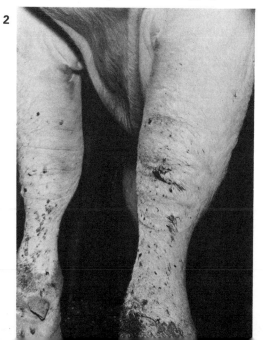

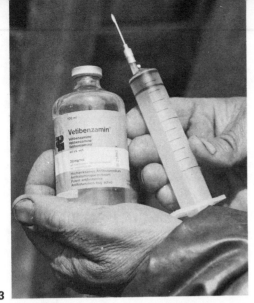

3

the same germ that causes summer mastitis. This germ is a normal resident of the tonsils of most cows, and every now and then the bug escapes into the bloodstream and travels down into the udder and into the lymph glands of the legs. In all these places the bug lies dormant, but nonetheless ever ready to multiply and grow when the resistance of the surrounding tissues is lowered sufficiently.

In this kind of 'big leg', what happens is

4

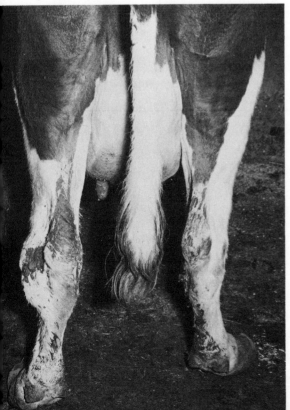

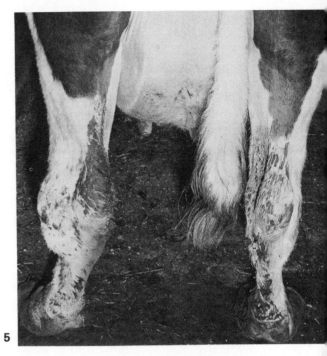

5

that first of all the leg, usually the outside of the hock, is bruised and damaged, either by the cow's persistent lying on hard bare floors or by her slipping and falling in the act of rising.

Usually the skin of the leg is not cut or broken. In fact it need not be, since the causal germ, the *C. pyogenes*, is already living inside the cow.

This bug invades the bruised tissue from the nearest gland, multiplies and grows, and in a comparatively short time produces a septic leg and a very sick cow which often has to be scrapped and replaced.

This condition becomes serious because the toxins or waste products from the multiplying *C. pyogenes* bugs not only produce pus, but also actually destroy the damaged tissue, so that in the resultant septic leg one not only has to deal with simple abscess formation, but also with fairly extensive areas of necrosis (*i.e.*, dead tissue).

This explains why lancing of the leg is so often ineffective. The knife fails because it is not possible to remove all the dead muscle, tendons and ligaments.

Predisposing Causes
Insufficient and unsuitable bedding, slippery floors, inadequate stall space and cubicles or beds that are too short. Any one of these defects in husbandry can cause a flare-up, though trouble is most likely where there is a combination of several of them.

Symptoms
These are unmistakable; the swelling usually starts at the hock and if untreated rapidly spreads up the leg (5).

Treatment
The first essential is to find out and remove the predisposing factor or factors because obviously if the leg bruising is going to continue, the patients are going to take more curing and recurrence will always be a possibility.

Medicinally, a course of three intramuscular injections of 10, 15 and 20 cc of *C. pyogenes* Toxoid or Vaccine at two-day intervals appears to work extremely well, provided treatment is started immediately the leg swelling appears.

Prevention
If cases keep coming, then obviously the predisposing factors just have to be eliminated, and I think this is far and away the most sensible way to tackle the problem.

Fortunately the widespread use of open yards and cubicles has done much to reduce the incidence.

3
Blackleg

THE sudden death of any heifer, bull or bullock under two years of age should be regarded with grave suspicion, especially if a blood examination proves negative for anthrax.

Cause
Blackleg (often called blackquarter or 'struck') is a gas gangrene affecting cattle and sheep and is caused by the growth of a germ called the *Clostridium chauvoei* in the muscles and surrounding tissues (1).

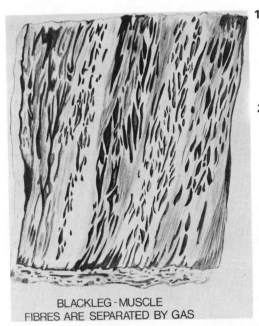

BLACKLEG - MUSCLE
FIBRES ARE SEPARATED BY GAS

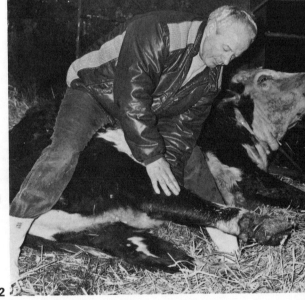

Symptoms
The *Clostridium chauvoei* sporulates like the anthrax bacillus and the Clostridial germ that causes tetanus. The blackleg spores can live for a long time on pastures and in the soil, and often pass through the digestive tracts of cattle and sheep.

It used to be thought that the germs travelled to the muscles from the intestine, but it is now fairly certain that the spores gain entry through a wound. The wound may not be large; in fact in cattle it is often not possible to detect one, but it is

139

more than likely that even minute wounds like fly bites can allow the spores to enter. The muscle in the vicinity of the wound becomes swollen and gaseous and feels as though tissue paper were under the skin instead of muscle (2).

Some scientists disagree with the wound infection explanation. They say that the *Clostridium chauvoei* lies dormant in the muscles until conditions become suitable for its growth. Personally I support wound infection theory every time. It is more logical and ties up with my own personal experience.

Blackleg is recognised as essentially a disease of permanent pastures and without doubt there are 'blackleg farms' and 'blackleg fields'. Unlike anthrax, the contamination of pastures is not due to the burying or neglect of infected carcases. It appears that the disease is perpetuated simply by the spores in the soil being maintained and increased by the constant pasturing of cattle and sheep.

Treatment
It can be treated provided it is diagnosed sufficiently early. Practically all the antibiotics are effective against the germ. The disease develops so rapidly, however, that only rarely does one catch it early enough.

Prevention
Obviously there is nothing that one can do to control blackleg from the pasture husbandry point of view. But fortunately extremely reasonably priced and highly efficient vaccines are available.

In cattle the vaccine should be injected when the animal is between three and six months old. A high degree of immunity develops in about ten days and appears to be sufficient in most cases to protect the animals completely though on 'blackleg farms' I recommend a booster dose of vaccine 6–12 months after the first.

4
Anthrax

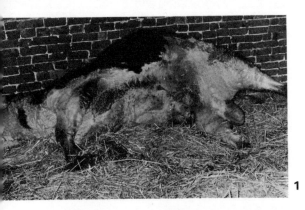

A DEAD cow, a dead bullock, a dead calf, the discovery of any one of these immediately fills us with an involuntary feeling of apprehension (1). What has caused the death? Could it be anthrax? At any rate, our consciences usually make us report the sudden death to the police or to the veterinary surgeon.

This is the correct procedure because sudden death could always be due to anthrax—anywhere and at any time.

Cause

Anthrax is caused by a germ called the *Bacillus anthracis* (2) which has the power to sporulate when exposed to the atmosphere, *i.e.*, it forms around itself a protective capsule which can guard it and keep it alive for many years.

This fact explains why there are certain fields where anthrax always seems to be a potential menace. Probably in years gone by, someone unwittingly shallow-buried one or several opened anthrax carcases.

The spores, from these carcases which have the power of propagation (all anthrax spores can multiply) have penetrated through the soil layers (by means of rising ground water or earthworms) to the surface to be picked up by grazing animals.

Drinking water passing over or through the anthrax fields can also carry the spores, and in warm weather particularly it can flare up infection.

Animals Affected

Cattle, sheep, horses, goats, pigs, mink,

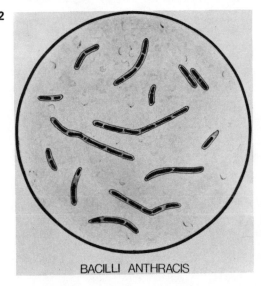

BACILLI ANTHRACIS

141

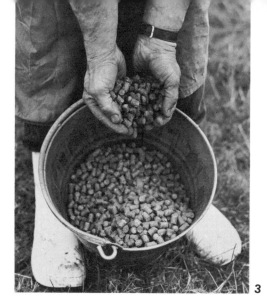

3

dogs, elephants, ostriches, deer, man, birds, wild animals, and even frogs and fish are all susceptible to anthrax.

Sources of Disease

Apart from the odd few anthrax fields, anthrax spores find their way into this country in imported foodstuffs (3). For this reason cattle are the most likely farm animals to become infected simply because they are more liable to eat the considerable number of spores required to flare up an infection.

Another possible, though less likely

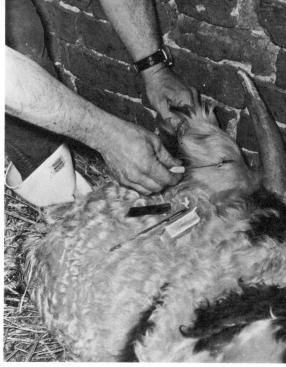

4

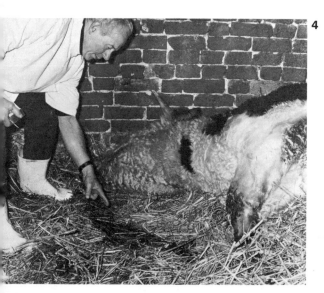

5

source, is the imported components of artificial manures. These have become contaminated chiefly by spores from the bones of affected carcases.

It is only rarely that anthrax is transmitted from one animal to another. When two or several cows in a herd are affected it is usually due to all of them having eaten a fatal number of spores more or less simultaneously. The bacilli do not generally invade the bloodstream until after death.

When eaten, the spores get into the animal's tonsils and travel via the body's drainage system to the intestines where they germinate into bacilli and produce their devastating effect.

6

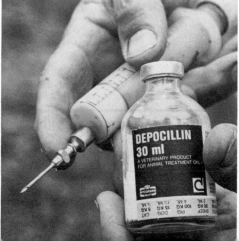

Symptoms

Symptoms may appear at any time from one to fourteen days after the spores are swallowed.

All anthrax cases don't die suddenly. In fact I have seen infected cattle ill for over three days.

The symptoms are those of general depression. The animal stands with hanging head and staring eye. The temperature is usually very high, though not always. In the three-days case I've just quoted, for example, the temperature remained subnormal.

The appetite is completely lost, and with the inappetence there is first of all constipation, and then diarrhoea—thin watery faeces usually mixed with blood.

Often large quantities of apparently pure blood are passed and a similar discharge may also pour from the mouth, nostrils (4) and vulva (all the natural openings). Death finally results usually in 24 to 48 hours, with signs of shivering, cramp and asphyxiation. It is not by any means pleasant to watch.

Usually, however, the animal is found dead. When this happens the correct procedure is to report the loss immediately either to your own veterinary surgeon or to the police. If to the police, in due course a veterinary inspector of the Ministry of Agriculture will appear, cut the small ear vein, take a blood smear and swab (5), prepare and stain his slides and examine them under a microscope.

If the result is positive, the carcase will have to be burned, but the local constable will organise this. Any labour provided by the farmer is fully chargeable to the local authority, as is any disinfectant, fuel or refreshment.

Treatment

Treatment is possible if it is applied early enough.

Modern antibiotics attack the *Bacillus anthracis* (6). Many of the high cattle fevers of unknown origin are quite probably due to anthrax, and the prompt response to antibiotic therapy (so often taken for granted) must have prevented very many deaths from anthrax.

Prevention

When I find a positive anthrax case I always advise the cutting down of the quantities of concentrates for a few days. I don't advise a change of food because, by the time the death occurs, it is practically certain that the entire herd will have already eaten some of the anthrax spores. Not only that, by eating the spores they will probably have immunised themselves fairly strongly against a future attack.

I recommend reducing the concentrates by 25 per cent for a period of 10 to 12 days. After that time the immunity should be established and it is then safe to resume normal feeding.

A vaccine is available but I don't think vaccination is worth while.

5
Other Causes of Sudden Death

APART from anthrax and blackleg (and hypomagnesaemia, of course) three other causes of sudden death should always be borne in mind—lightning stroke, electrocution and yew tree poisoning.

(a) Lightning Stroke

This is a comparatively common condition. Seldom does a thunderstorm occur without reports of deaths. Sometimes the cow or cows are found lying under a tree or alongside a wire fence though more often than not the victim is found in the open field (1).

Symptoms

If the animal is alive after being struck (and this happens only occasionally), the symptoms are those of spinal damage, that is, partial or complete paralysis and hyperexcitability; single marks may or may not be seen along the back, shoulder or leg.

If, as is usual, the animal is dead, single marks can usually be detected, but in most

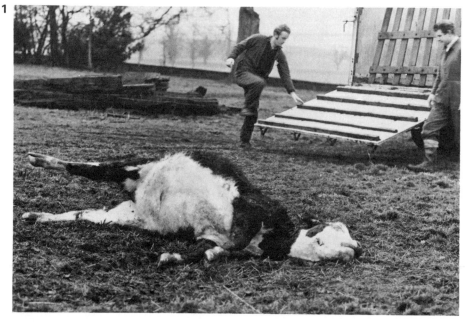

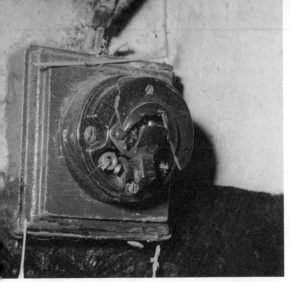

2

cases the diagnosis has to be confirmed by post-mortem examination of the carcase and this is very much a job for a veterinary surgeon.

Post-mortem Signs
Acute congestion and minute haemorrhages throughout both lungs and often strings of partially clotted blood in the windpipe and bronchi.

The heart is contracted, with the main pumping cavities—the ventricles—nearly always empty.

The blood is not 'fluid', as so many text books say, though if the post-mortem examination is carried out quickly, some of the blood is not clotted, and even after a day or two the clots are soft and nothing like as clearly formed as when death is due to other causes.

Sometimes a wad of grass is in the mouth, but the rest of the digestive system is absolutely normal with no signs of bloat. In fact I have never seen a bloated rumen (first stomach) in a case of true lightning stroke.

Close examination will usually reveal single marks on the skin surface on the shoulder, back or occasionally on the legs.

Under the hide the corresponding areas are clearly and distinctly marked by extensive bruising and haemorrhages. These marks are continued into the tissues under the skin and deep into the muscles, with occasionally the acute damage following into and even right through the chest and abdomen.

It has been my experience that it is easy to give an absolute positive diagnosis of lightning stroke provided the post-mortem examination can be carried out within 24 hours of death.

(b) Electrocution

This condition I have seen on a number of occasions during my thirty-odd years in agricultural practice. In fact I well remember one morning around 6 am being called to a herd of sixty cows, three of which lay dead while most of the others were bawling their heads off and dancing or staggering about the cowshed. It wasn't a pleasant experience.

Cause
A fault in the electrical system which can usually be traced to a broken switch or a chewed wire (2).

Symptoms
The symptoms are as I have described them and the diagnosis is usually confirmed when one of the 'live' stalls is accidentally touched by an attendant.

Treatment
Shocked animals which are not dead should be given antihistamine injections.

Post-mortem Lesions
The general picture is similar to lightning stroke though the singe marks are absent and the tissue bruising is nothing like so severe as in lightning stroke.

(c) Yew Tree Poisoning

In cattle yew is the most rapidly fatal of all plant poisons. I have seen twenty cattle lying dead under a yew tree within hours of their gaining access to the danger area.

The symptoms are sudden death and there is no known antidote to the poison.

Obviously, therefore, it is vitally essential never to allow cattle anywhere near yew trees.

6
Bracken Poisoning

BRACKEN can be present and readily accessible on a farm for many years without apparently causing any harm. Without warning, often in *the early spring* when the bracken shoots have reached a succulent stage of growth (1), the cattle suddenly develop a taste for the bracken. The results can be disastrous.

Symptoms

The most general typical symptom is blood-stained diarrhoea. The animal runs a temperature of around 104° to 106° F and there may be a swelling in the throat region. Occasionally there may be a bloody discharge from the mouth or nostrils (2).

The blood comes from small haemorrhages which may occur all over the body but especially in the intestines, lungs, and occasionally in the more superficial

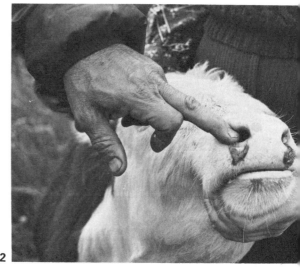

mucous membranes (hence the nose-bleeding). These haemorrhages allow secondary bacteria to move in and 'take over'. This 'invasion' not only makes treatment much more difficult, but often means that an animal can die or develop severe symptoms a considerable time after taking in the original poison.

Treatment

Obviously this has to be aimed at controlling the secondary invaders as well as attempting to combat the poison and heal the damaged tissues. A heavy umbrella of antibiotics has to be provided for a considerable time, and large doses of vitamins B and K are used.

A drug called DL-Batyl Alcohol has been tried with some success. This drug appears to prevent, to some extent, the damage to the blood corpuscles which the poisonous component of the bracken normally causes.

The antibiotics and vitamins have to be given simultaneously.

Prevention

The answer to bracken poisoning is obvious and simple, that is, remove the source. The best way to do this is by repeated cutting of the plants combined with solid grazing of the area. Bracken sufferers should never forget that it is the succulent shoots of the bracken which contain the virulent poison. Stubble of cut bracken is never dangerous. The repeated cutting combined with the intensive grazing will never allow the plant to become a source of trouble.

GENERAL ADVICE

1
How to Lift a Cow

ONE of the commonest nightmares among herdsmen is the cow unable to rise after calving (1). Usually it is the sequel of milk fever, the partial paralysis being due to injured nerves or joints caused by splaying on a slippery floor. Hypomagnesaemia and aphosphorosis are other common predisposing causes.

In heifers the injuries are usually the result of excessive pulling on that first calf.

But, whatever the cause, such a case means a frustrating heart-breaking task of prolonged nursing, quite apart from a great deal of inconvenience. And the question often arises as to whether or not treatment is worth while.

Many and varied have been the methods employed in the past to try to lift the cow. Until comparatively recently all failed simply because any pressure on the floor of a cow's chest or belly resulted in loss of power in the legs.

1

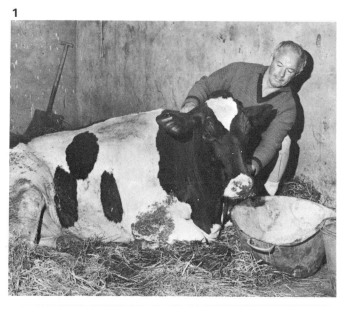

However, there is now in the possession **2**
of most veterinary surgeons an American
invention called the 'Bagshaw Hoist' (2)
which fits on to and exerts its pressure on
the pin bones of the pelvis. This apparatus
makes treatment not only economical, but
also highly successful.

The 'Bagshaw Hoist' is made of light
steel alloy and is simple in design with
two hinged 'wings' that can be closed
under pressure by a cross bar and screw.
There is a looped swivelled handle at the
top.

I personally have saved many cows' lives **3**
with this hoist, and the object of this series
of pictures is to demonstrate the technique
and to show how successful it can be even
when, as was the case with the animal
photographed, she has been down for a
good many days.

The first job is to remove the bedding
from the floor below and in front of the
cow (3). This is because such bedding is
soiled and wet and the floor underneath
is usually as slippery as the ice on a
skating rink.

Next, sand or grit is sprinkled over the
floor surface (4) so that subsequently,
when the debilitated cow is lifted, she will
be less likely to slip down again. This
should be done in all cases where a cow
is down and unable to rise.

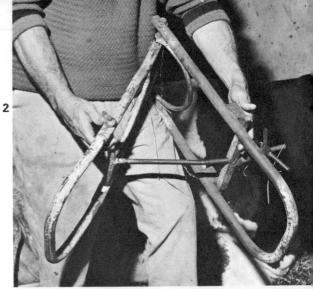

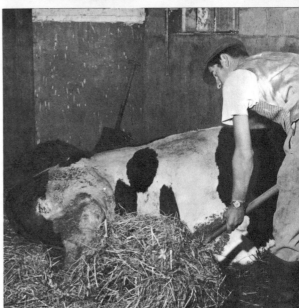

4

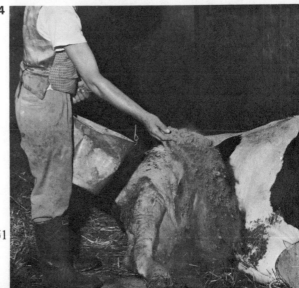

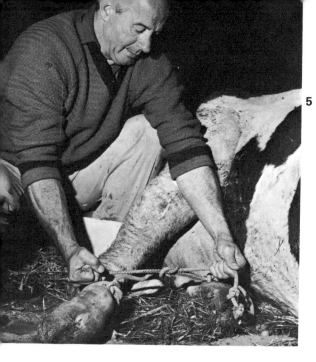

5   Now probably the most important thing of all. The hind legs are hobbled, *i.e.,* tied together just above the fetlocks by two short lengths of rope, leaving a space of approximately 18 inches between the legs (5). In tying the ropes around the fetlocks and to each other a reef knot is always used. (This is illustrated here very clearly.) This hobbling prevents further splaying and the cow can stand and walk with the hobbles in position.

Another very important point—the cow's head is haltered since it is vital to have her head firmly held during lifting to avoid 'plunging' (6).

Fitting the hoist. The picture (7) illustrates exactly how the lower curvatures of the wings are fitted over the cow's pin bones. The cross bar is screwed up firmly but not excessively tightly. If the hoist is too uncomfortable it may stop the cow making the effort to stand on her own.

6

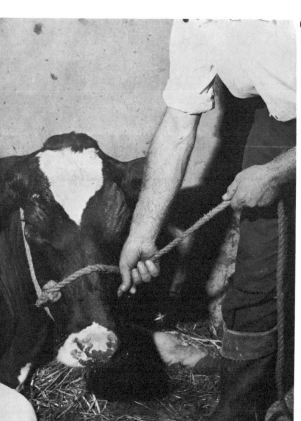

7

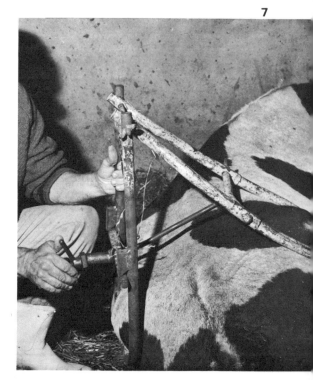

A strong block and tackle is now hooked **8**
to a double or triple rope loop around the
highest beam obtainable above the cow
(8). A chain block and tackle is the ideal,
though I have often lifted cattle successfully with a rope set.

The lower hook of the tackle is fitted
on to the hoist handle (9).

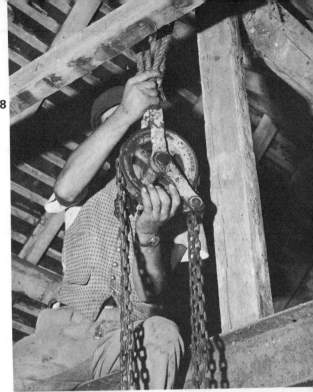

9

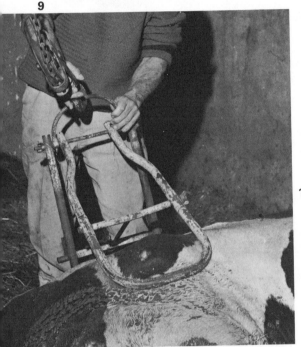

With two assistants, one holding the
head rigidly and one keeping the block
chain in the right groove, the hind-
quarters are lifted up (10).

10

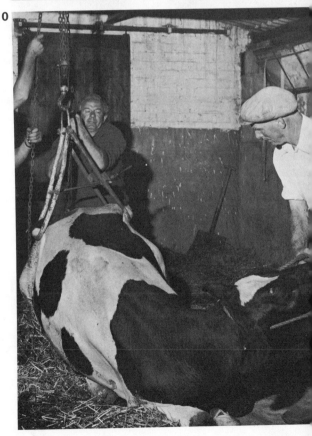

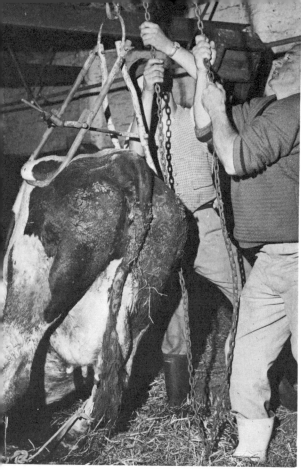

11   Three parts of the way up (11)— and a dangerous time for 'plunging'. On no account must the head be let go at this stage.

The cow has struggled forward and is taking her weight on all four legs, so the hoist is now released and removed. Note how the rope hobbles have stopped the hind legs from splaying (12).

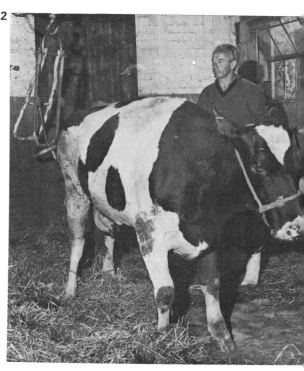

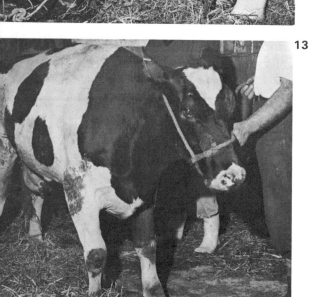

The cow is up and has moved a step forward. But her knees are rubbed raw with bed sores—in fact any further damage could expose the joints (13).

The bed sores are cleansed and powdered

over with a combined sulphur and anti-biotic dusting powder (14).

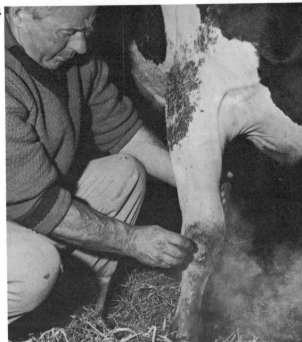

The damaged knees are bound up and protected by cotton wool and elastic adhesive bandages (15).

The sight that every afflicted herdsman

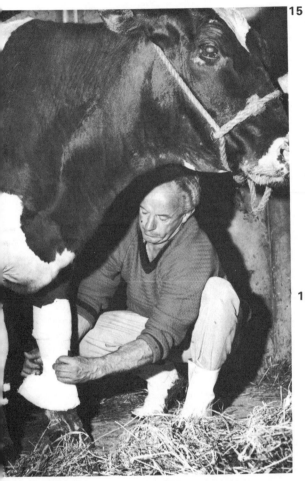

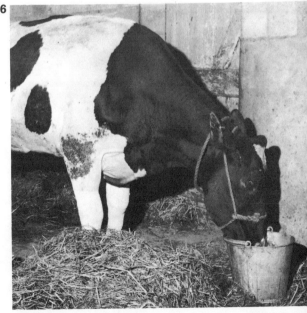

dreams about—a cow, down for a long time, now up, standing correctly and moving forward for a drink of water (16).

2
How to Turn a Cow Over

WHEN a cow is down and unable to rise it is extremely important that she should be turned over on her other side. Such a condition may arise in an acute attack of milk fever. It may also occur in phosphorus deficiency, staggers, or debility and injury following a difficult calving.

In the case of an acute milk fever, turning the cow over on her other side will often save her life by alleviating the blown-up condition which prevails.

With all the other cases, repeated turning at least twice a day will be necessary to avoid bed sores and give the animal the maximum chance of recovery.

The simplest and most effective turnover technique is as follows:

First of all, take a good length of strong rope and make a running noose at one end (1).

1

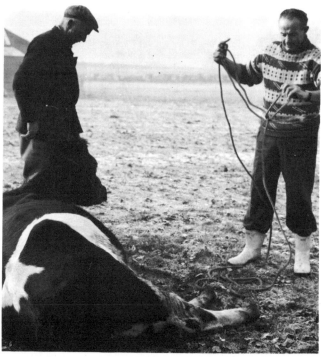

Fix the running noose on the upper leg immediately below the fetlock (2). It is permissible to fix the rope above the fetlock, but when this is done, sometimes the noose slips up the leg and loses its effectiveness.

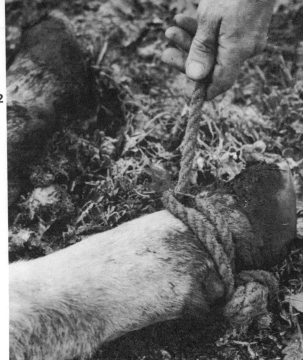

Now pass the centre part of the rope underneath the head, brisket and both knees of the animal (3). By pulling the rope to and fro with the aid of an assistant, work it back underneath the cow's body. For this job the assistant can be a wife or even a small child, or in an emergency the job can be done by the man alone.

Continue adjusting the rope until it

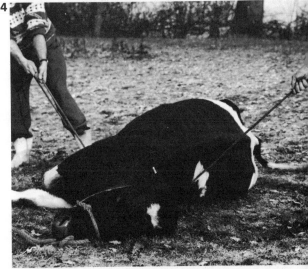

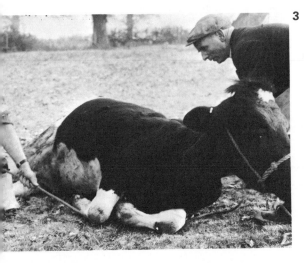

reaches approximately the centre of the animal's back (4).

Now get the assistant to steady the cow's head and whilst he's doing so pull the rope through as far as possible (5), thus bringing the tied foot close up underneath the abdomen.

Next throw the free end of the rope over the cow's back to the opposite side (6).

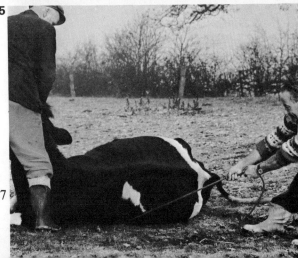

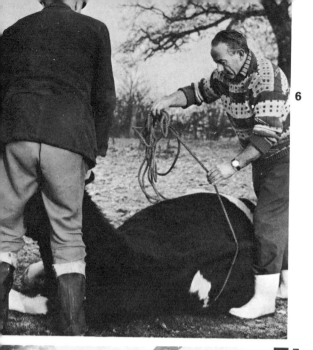

6

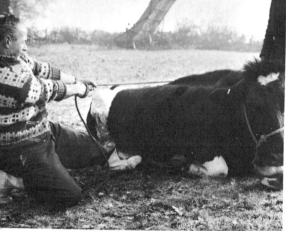

7

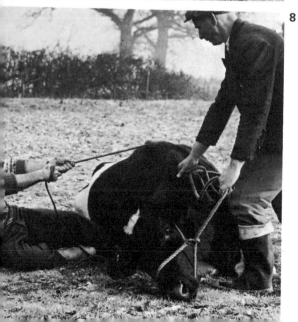

8

Using the tied foot as a fulcrum, pull the cow into a sitting position (7).

Then pull her bodily over (8).

This picture (9) shows the new position of the tied foot.

9

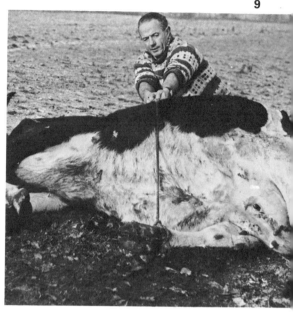

Finally, sit the animal on to her brisket, remove the rope and the job is done (10). In most cases the cow will be so relieved she will sit herself up with no bother.

10

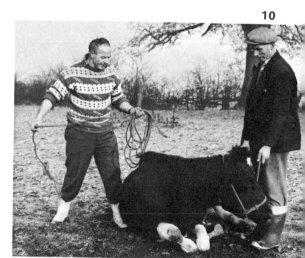

3
How to Pare the Feet

FIRST, the tools for the job.

Every farmer should provide himself with a decent set of knives and a pair of really first-class clippers.

He will also need a stout wooden bar covered over with one or two sacks wound round and tied with binder twine, a decent length of strong rope, and a bale of straw (1).

Method of Restraint

For a bull, a halter to augment the ring is usually all that is necessary (2).

If, however, the bull is fractious or if the patient is a cow, then a running noose should be made round the base of the horn (or around the neck in the case of hornless cattle). The free end of the rope should now be brought down the front of the face and a half-hitch made around the lower jaw (3).

This will give considerable purchase and

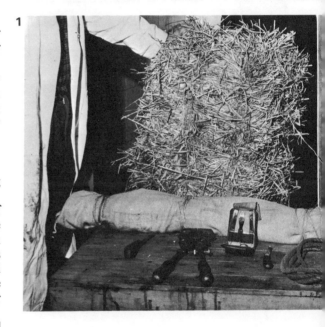

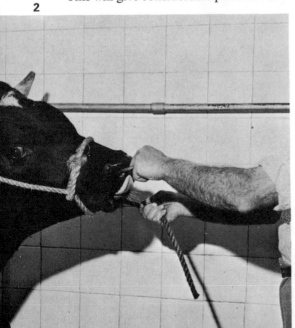

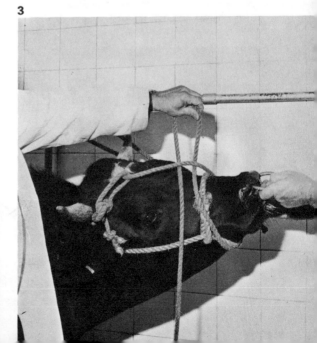

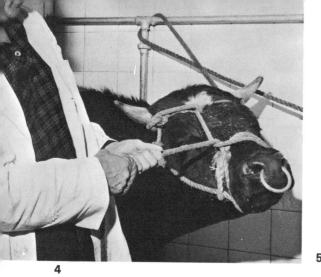

4

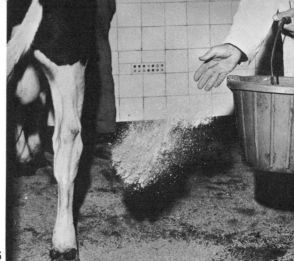

5

will make restraint very much easier. It is essential, during a long spell of working at the feet, that the cow's or bull's head should be held rigidly (4).

The Floor

Always, before starting to clip feet, spread plenty of sand or grit underneath the hind feet. Sawdust is an ideal bedding to use and the sawdust can be spread on top of the sand (5).

How To Lift A Hind Foot

(a) With the Bar

With a quiet cow or docile bull the padded bar may be all that is necessary. The bar bears in the angle of the hock and each assistant helps to steady the back-end by pressing his shoulder tightly against the animal (6).

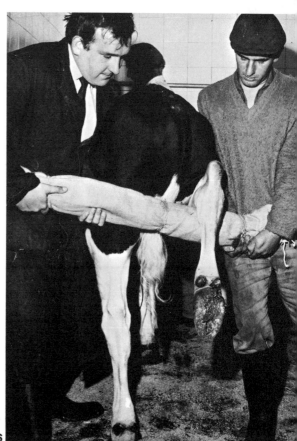

6

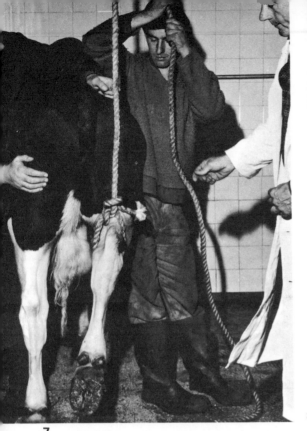

7

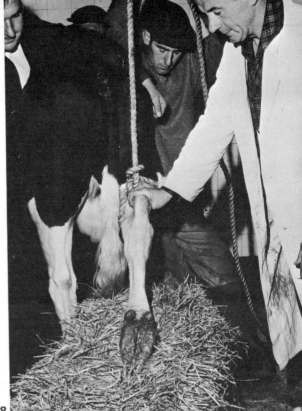

8

(b) With the Rope

For most foot-clipping jobs, it is better to use a thick rope. Tie a reef knot *above* the hock and pass the free end over a roof beam (7).

The bale of straw can now be put length-ways underneath the foot to take most of the weight (8).

How To Lift A Front Foot

Tie the rope, again using a reef knot, around the coronet and pass the free end of the rope over the top of the animal's shoulder to the other side (9). When the foot is lifted, the assistant stands on the opposite side and pulls downward on the rope so that the weight of the leg is taken chiefly by the animal's shoulders and back.

The bale can again be used underneath the foot. Fortunately the forefeet rarely require extensive clipping.

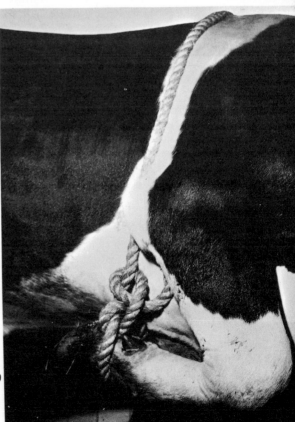

9

161

The Technique of Clipping

The most important thing to bear in mind in clipping a cow's or bull's foot is that the toes should be clipped as short as possible and the heels left as long as possible (10–11).

Clipping the wall, however, is not enough. *It is essential that the underside of the sole should be made concave and this is where the sharp knives come in* (12). When the toes of a cow or bull become exceptionally long, the animal is thrown back on the heels and the under surface of the sole becomes overgrown, convex and consequently subject to bruising. The bruises have to be cut out and the foot left so that the wall is higher than the sole.

The Finished Foot

With the toes short, heels long, bruises cut out, and the sole concave and below the level of the wall (13).

If at any time during the clipping, the 'quick' is cut by mistake, then a powerful antiseptic spray should be used and the foot should be covered over for two or three days.

10

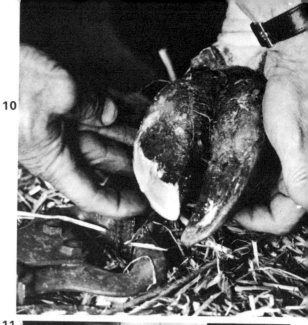

11

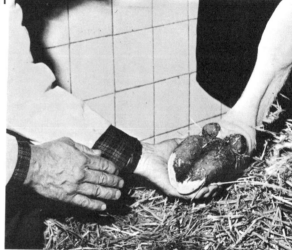

12

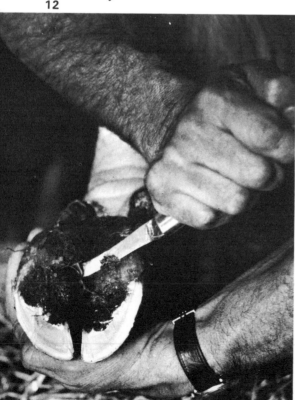

13

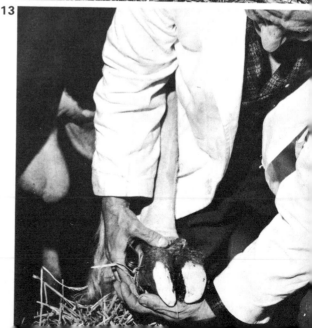

4
How to Ring a Bull

RINGING a bull is a comparatively simple task. Nevertheless if not done correctly, secondary sepsis may set in and death can result.

Tools For The Job
A stout rope with a fixed noose on one end: a clean pair of bullringing forceps: a ring and screw: and most important of all a bottle of antiseptic and some cotton wool (1).

Securing The Head
Make a running noose by passing the end of the rope through the fixed noose and get an assistant to steady the bull's head (2).

Put the running noose around the base of the horns and tighten it with the fixed noose in the centre of the poll (3).

1

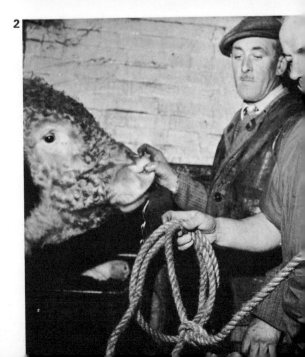

2

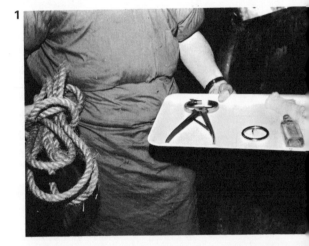

3

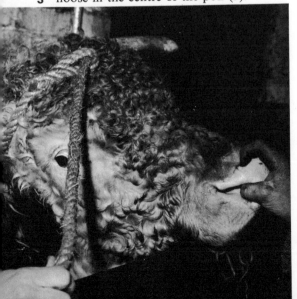

Now bring the free end of the rope **4**
down the centre of the face and, holding
the rope about 6″ from the nostril, loop
the free end under both jaws (4).

Now bring the free end up and underneath the face part of the rope thus
forming a 'half-hitch' (5).

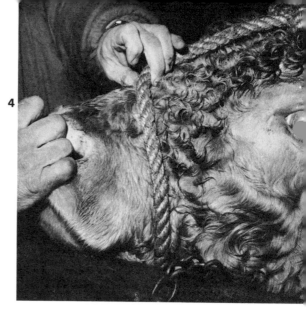

5

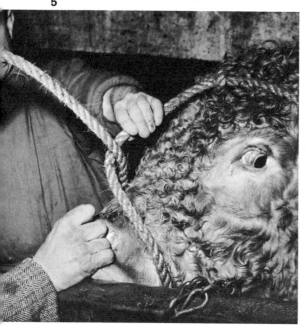

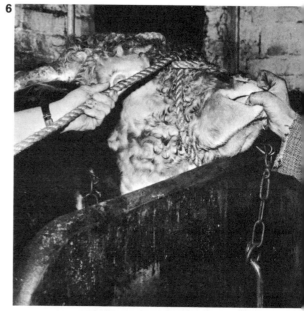

6

The bull's head can now be pulled round
to the side and if it hasn't been possible
for the nose to be held during the roping
the 'half-hitch' will enable the head to be
lifted and pulled round (6).

With the rope thus fixed, the assistant
can pull the head over the stall (7) or if the
bull is in a box over the top of a half door. **7**

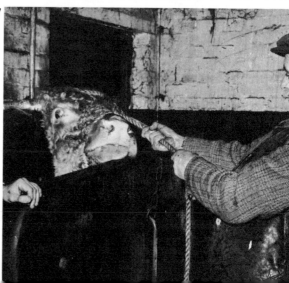

164

If the bull is dehorned, the running noose should be passed over the head and around the neck but the centre part of the noose should be brought down approximately 6″ from the poll; this prevents the rope tightening around the neck and causing a choking sensation which would make the bull plunge and struggle (8).

A useful hint to secure the head is to pass the end of the rope through the anchor of the neighbouring cow-tie or around any similar fixture (9).

Inserting The Ring

No matter how apparently clean the bull-ringing forceps may be, the punch should be soaked thoroughly in a powerful non-irritant antiseptic (10). This strict asepsis is essential to prevent infection.

The punch is inserted, blunt end first, into the nostril and moved forward

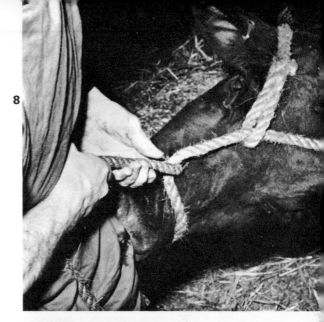

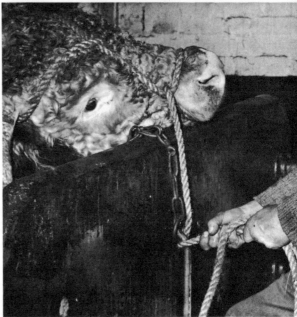

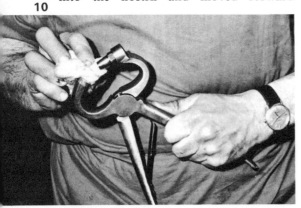

approximately 1″ (11). This ensures that the hole will be punched through the nasal cartilage and not through the more tender nasal septum which lies between the cartilage and the skin of the nostril. *This is a very important point in bull-ringing, because if the septum is pierced instead of the cartilage, the nose will remain tender for a considerable time and the bull will resent strongly the handling of the ring. Also when the septum is pierced, infection is more likely to arise.*

When the punch is closed tightly it is a good idea to move its head to and fro

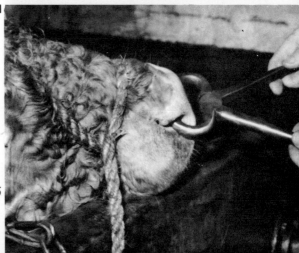

165

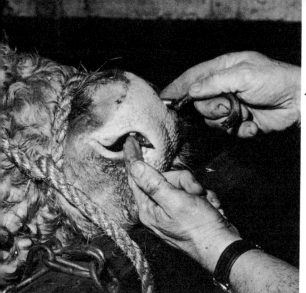

12 once or twice to make sure that the hole is punched cleanly.

Another important point is to coat the ring with a powerful non-irritant antiseptic. Some veterinary surgeons advise boiling the ring before use; this is an excellent idea, but not always practicable.

Now guide the sharp point of the ring through the hole with the index finger of the left hand (12). Again this is a useful hint because if you poke about blindly looking for the hole, the bull will struggle violently.

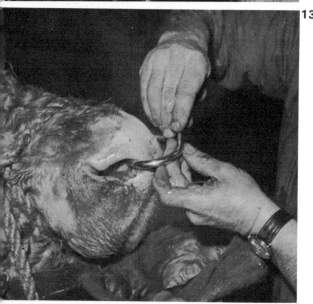

13 An old tip well worth taking is to hold a cap or hat underneath while 'screwing up' in case the screw drops and is lost in the bedding (13). This is advisable even with the modern type of screw.

Finally, the ring should be again coated with antiseptic (14).

14

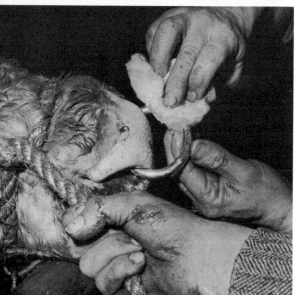

5
Needle Know-How

IT is essential to know the correct way to take care of and to use syringes and needles on the farm.

The Syringe and Its Care

The best syringe is of nylon with a metal ending to fit the needle. It lasts longer than a glass syringe and stands up to any amount of misuse. A 20 c.c. or 10 c.c. size will serve for cattle, sheep and pigs. In addition to the syringe, you need a flutter valve (1) for injecting large quantities of fluid (for, say, calcium borogluconate in milk fever case).

Two sizes of needle are necessary—$\frac{1}{2}''$ and $1\frac{1}{2}''$ long (2). They should be stainless steel, strong and reasonably thick. When the points become blunt, throw them away and replace them.

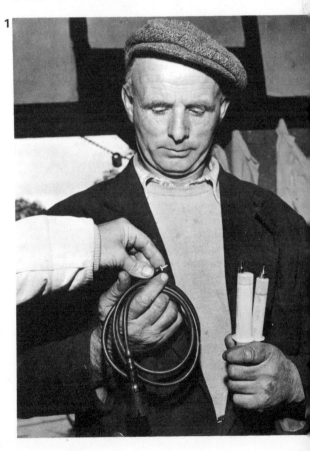

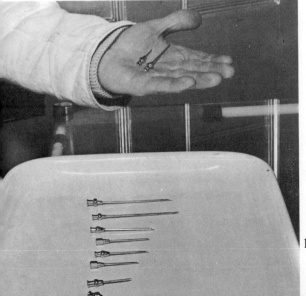

Wrong (3). He's going to boil the syringe with the plunger in position. Always take the syringe to pieces. Boil the entire kit once a month. In between times, keep in a cold steriliser.

Cold sterilisation is simply keeping the kit immersed in an instrument antiseptic. Your veterinary surgeon will supply you with the correct antiseptic solution (4).

How To Make a Subcutaneous Injection

The correct site for subcutaneous (*i.e.,*

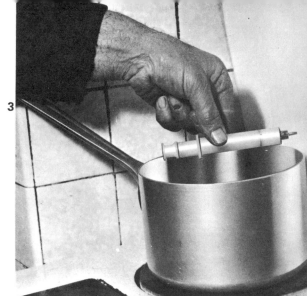

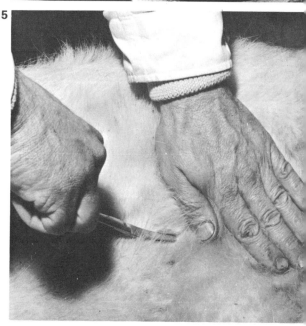

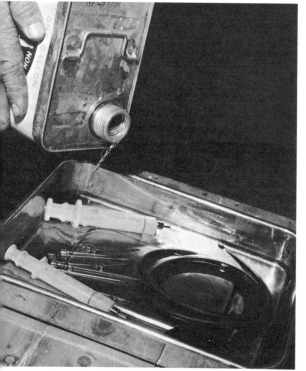

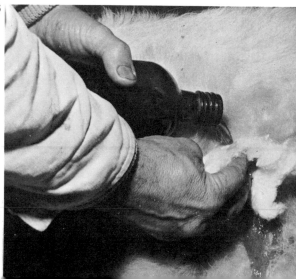

under the skin) injection is one hand's breadth behind the ridge of the cow's shoulder (5). Clip the hair around the site and swab it with a powerful skin antiseptic (6). Your veterinary surgeon will supply you with the correct fluid.

It is important to put the injection fluid under the skin and not into the underlying tissues, or a huge lump will develop. To get the needle inserted, correctly hold a fold of the skin in the hand directly above the site. You will hear the air being sucked

168

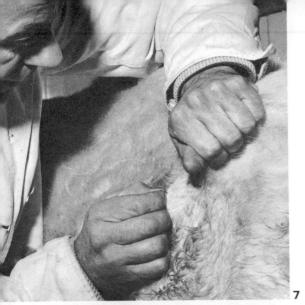

7

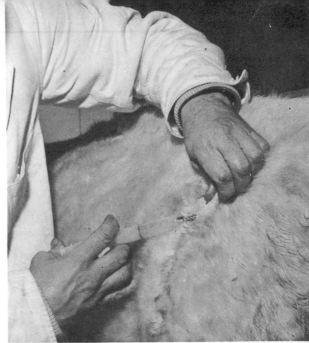

8

in through the needle when the needle point is correctly placed (7).

In subcutaneous injections always insert the needle without the syringe attached. When fitting the syringe hold the fold of skin in the hand over the site to make sure the needle doesn't penetrate too far (8).

How To Use The Flutter Valve
With the flutter valve it is vitally important to have the needle point only underneath the skin, because of the large quantities of fluid usually injected (9).

The most important point of all in flutter valve injections is rub the injection site thoroughly after every injection (10). Make certain the fluid is dispersed over a large area underneath the skin otherwise you will get irritation, and abscess, and an unholy mess.

How To Give An Intramuscular Injection
The correct site for an intramuscular injection is one hand's breadth in front of

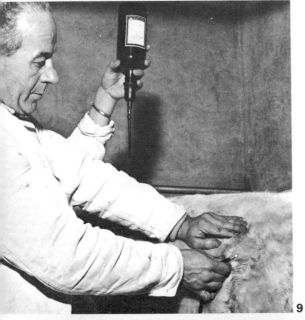

9

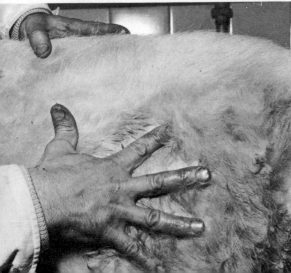

10

the ridge of the shoulder joint, *i.e.,* on the side of the neck (11).

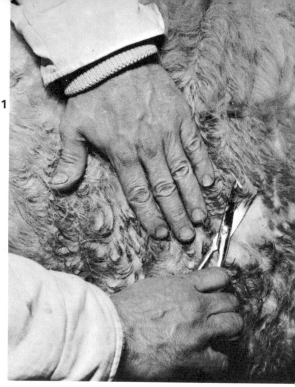

Always use the 1½″ needle for an intramuscular injection. Unless the fluid is injected fairly deeply in the muscles, swellings and abscesses will result. Don't be afraid to thrust the needle straight in to its full length for an intramuscular dose (12).

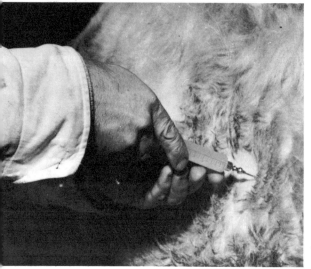

It is important never to use the muscles at the top of the cow's hind-quarters (13), because if ever you get abscess formation in this area you can't get proper drainage and the cow will finish up in the knacker's yard.

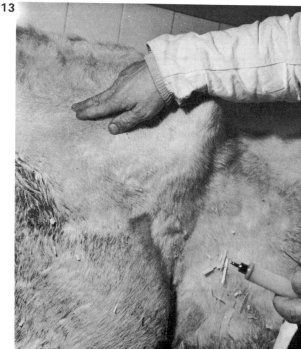

INDEX

Index